FACES OF COMBAT
PTSD and TBI

Also by Eric Newhouse
available from EricNewhouse.com and Issues Press

Alcohol: Cradle to Grave

Nearly Knighted: Life after Winning a Pulitzer Prize

FACES OF COMBAT
PTSD and TBI

One Journalist's Crusade
to Improve Treatment
for Our Veterans

Eric Newhouse

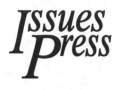 An imprint of Idyll Arbor, Inc.
39129 264th Ave SE, Enumclaw, WA 98022

Cover design: Pat Kenny
Editor: Kenneth A. Lucas

Newhouse, Eric, 1945-
 Faces of combat, PTSD and TBI : join one man's battle to improve treatment for our veterans / Eric Newhouse.
    p. ; cm.
 Includes index.
 ISBN 978-1-930461-06-2 (alk. paper)
 1. Post-traumatic stress disorder--United States. 2. Veterans--Mental health care--United States. 3. Brain damage--United States. I. Title.
 [DNLM: 1. Health Services Needs and Demand--United States. 2. Veterans--United States. 3. Brain Injuries--United States. 4. Combat Disorders--United States. 5. Health Services Accessibility--United States. 6. Stress Disorders, Post-Traumatic--United States.
 WA 360 N548f 2008]
 RC552.P67N47 2008
 616.85'21--dc22
                                                            2008030462

ISBN 9781-930461-06-2

This book is gratefully dedicated

to the courageous combat vets and their families who shared their stories with me in the hope of helping their comrades and forcing reform of the system;

to the Great Falls Tribune, *which allows me to report on significant social issues; and*

to God, without whom none of this could have been possible.

◊ ◊ ◊

Jesus said to him, "'You shall love the Lord your God with all your heart, with all your soul, and with all your mind.'

This is the great and foremost commandment.

And the second is like it: 'You shall love your neighbor as yourself.'

On these two commandments depend the whole Law and the Prophets."

— Matthew 22:37-40

Contents

Preface

I was drafted into the U.S. Army in 1968 at the beginning of the war in Vietnam. A fresh graduate of the University of Wisconsin and a cub reporter for the Rockford (Illinois) *Morning Star*, I didn't want to go to Vietnam. I feared I would die there and I didn't want to die. U.S. Senator George McGovern of South Dakota was galvanizing a protest movement against the war; he was a hero to my generation, although I didn't get to know him personally until a decade later when I was working for the Associated Press in Pierre, South Dakota. In the late '60s, there were protest marches on campuses across America — Wisconsin was typically in the vanguard — and some young men went to Canada to avoid the draft. That was something I considered, but I could not bring myself to disobey the law. Instead, I told my wife-to-be that if Uncle Sam sent me home in a box with a flag draped over it, I wanted her to burn the flag.

As it happened, I never went to 'Nam. Through some glorious good fortune, I ended up as a writer on the base newspaper at Fort Meade, Maryland, and then as a public relations specialist for the U.S. Army Field Band and Soldiers Chorus, also based at Fort Meade.

Many of my friends were sent to fight, however, and not all of them came home. Over the years, most of them suffered and at least one committed suicide. I watched them, not really understanding what they were going through, and never asking the right questions. And I never knew how the war could affect even those who didn't fight in it.

About a decade ago, my youngest daughter, Sarah, graduated from Shepherd College just outside of Washington, DC. I was (and still am) the projects editor for the Great Falls (Montana) *Tribune*, and my wife Susie and I went back east for the graduation. I stayed with my daughter in DC over the Memorial Day weekend, and the veterans on Harleys who call themselves "Rolling Thunder" were everywhere. Squadrons of motorcycles were roaring up and down Pennsylvania Avenue, and I realized that it was the perfect opportunity to visit the Vietnam Veterans Memorial.

So we joined the line of burly bikers in their black leather jackets and inched forward until we came to that wall, containing the names of 58,000 soldiers who died in Vietnam, panel after panel after panel of them. I was looking at the wall, trying to figure out which two years of it I had served in the Army, when a park ranger came by. I asked whether one particular panel would commemorate those who had died at the end of 1969, and the ranger told me that this was indeed the panel.

"So," I said, turning to Sarah, "these panels would have been some of the soldiers I served with."

"Welcome home, sir," said the ranger.

Instantly, I was sobbing helplessly on my daughter's shoulder while the park ranger rubbed my shoulders. I couldn't believe it, still can't believe it. How could I have such an emotional reaction when I had never been in combat, never been shot at, never been forced to take a human life?

War scars us all, but does the most damage to those closest to it.

When the invasion of Iraq/Afghanistan was ordered by President George W. Bush, I began to sense the eerie echoes of Vietnam all over again. The only real difference was that there was no universal draft. Instead, the government began using what it called private security contractors, former soldiers fighting as mercenaries at about triple the pay of regular soldiers. As soldiers left the military to get rich as mercenaries, about a third of the forces in the field were contractors. It has been terribly expensive, but it avoided the draft that brought the pain of war home to all American families — and it avoided most of the huge protests, too.

So perhaps you can consider this book my protest. I want you to see war through the eyes of those who have been there. I want you to understand what it's like to come home, emotional warriors in a civilian world. And I want you to feel their frustration as the treatment that they deserve and need too often gets lost in bureaucratic paperwork.

As a journalist over the past four decades, I've tried to amplify the voices of those who usually go unheard so that the public and the policymakers understand what's happening to the people they don't see and to the people they're conditioned not to hear. Instead of showing the average, I deliberately want you to see the faces of those making extreme cries for help.

Because the reality is that many vets, even those who aren't extreme cases, aren't getting the help they need and deserve.

◊ ◊ ◊

In addition, I want you to know how war harms the combatants. Many of the experts, including those in the Department of Defense (DOD), say that 25 to 40 percent of the soldiers who come back from war will experience post-traumatic stress disorder (PTSD) so severely that they may require treatment, primarily counseling and medications, for many years, if not for the rest of their lives.

Between 2001 and the end of 2007, America has deployed 1.6 million troops into Iraq and Afghanistan. "Fifteen to 20 percent of OIF/OEF [Operation Iraqi Freedom/Operation Enduring Freedom] veterans will suffer from a diagnosable mental health disorder," said the VA's Special Committee on PTSD. "Another 15 to 20 percent may be at risk for significant symptoms short of full diagnosis, but severe enough to cause significant functional impairment." The Dole-Shalala Commission put the risk even higher: "Fifty-six percent of active duty, 60 percent of reserve component, and 76 percent of retired/separated service members say they have reported mental health symptoms to a health care provider."

Dr. James Peake, as of this writing the secretary of Veterans Affairs, thinks those estimates are too high. He told me: "About 30 percent of those coming back have some need for counseling, but it would not be appropriate to label them all with PTSD. We're still sorting out what percentage should be labeled with PTSD, but I think it's less than 30 percent."

A few months after I spoke with Dr. Peake, the RAND Corporation issued a 500-page report showing that one combat vet in three would come home with either PTSD, traumatic brain injury (TBI), or major depression. And it called those prevalence rates *conservative*.

That's a staggering number in itself, but most combat vets still think the problem is being understated. Some of the vets say that all who serve in combat will come home disabled, and that it would be better to reverse the assumption and offer help to *everyone* — let those who don't need it demonstrate that they don't.

◊ ◊ ◊

I also want you to understand how hard it is to get treatment. According to the Congressional Budget Office, nearly half the Iraqi/Afghan vets are eligible for help from the Veterans Administration because they've separated from active duty or because they are eligible as members of the Reserves or National Guard. They've been promised two years of free medical treatment for any service-related disability, but only about one-third of those seeking VA medical care since 2002 (for a variety of reasons) have actually been able to get it.

In 2008, the number of vets receiving treatment is expected to grow to 5.8 million as the 'Nam vets get older and the Iraqi/Afghan vets begin to realize their injuries. But the system is overloaded even without the Iraqi/Afghan vets.

"We saw 400,000 people with PTSD last year," VA secretary Peake told me early in 2008. "But it was a significantly smaller number from OIF/OEF. We had lots of Vietnam vets and some from World War II. It looks like we only had 37,000 PTSD cases from confirmed service in OIF/OEF."

Compare that 37,000 to the 480,000 predicted to have PTSD, TBI, or other significant health needs (30% of 1.6 million) and you can see that the VA will be overwhelmed if it doesn't more than double its current capacity.

It's frustratingly hard for a vet to get help. The Government Accountability Office (GAO) has found that the VA is so underfunded and understaffed that nearly half of the returning vets eligible for treatment did not receive it. The VA has an average delay of 177 days before it begins providing disability pay and benefits. And despite intensive review by the GAO, eight congressional committees, a presidential task force, a presidential commission, as well as the Pentagon and the VA itself, the government has no apparent solution.

It's only going to get worse unless we commit the necessary resources to solve the problem.

◊ ◊ ◊

Finally I want you to look at some of the possible solutions. Innovative programs, increased spending on effective resources, and improved treatments are all possible ways out of this crisis. It's not hopeless, but we do need to step up and decide to take care of our veterans.

◊ ◊ ◊

I'd like to thank the Great Falls *Tribune* and particularly its publisher, Jim Strauss, for allowing me to use stories I wrote for the *Tribune* in this book. I'd also like to thank my wife Susie for her good suggestions on writing this book and my good friend Paul Edwards for reading a rough draft of it and telling me how to make it better. Joe Califano, chairman of the National Center for Addiction and Substance Abuse at Columbia University, and CASA's vice-president Sue Foster also invited me to sit in on a very useful conference on stress and alcoholism in New York City. Finally, local counselors like Christine Krupar King, Keli Remus, and Dr. Michael Mason have been invaluable in suggesting PTSD victims for me to talk to and helping me understand what they were saying.

You will notice throughout the book that I discuss the situation in Montana more than the rest of the country. There are reasons for that. The simple reason is that Montana is where I live. The complicated part is that we are looking at men and women who have severe emotional injuries from their military service. I didn't call them on the phone for a quick half-hour chat. I spent *days* with many of them before they trusted me with their stories. But don't worry, you can find the same Faces of Combat in your own community. And every single one of them needs our help.

Part 1
The Problem

Here we look at the Faces of Combat to see what happened to them in the service of our country, how they were treated when they returned, and the ways our country has either helped them or tossed them aside.

- 1 -
Death makes a difference

If many of the Faces of Combat look tormented, it's because they came home laden with guilt and shame. Montanans recognized that for the first time after March 4, 2007, when one combat vet put a .22 against his head, muffled it with a comforter, and ended his life as quietly as a book drops. He had PTSD and didn't get the help he needed.

Montana has always been a very patriotic state, drawing recruits from prairie towns and from its Indian reservations. It ranks tops among the states with the greatest number of vets per capita, and it prides itself on caring for its soldiers and their families.

That's why it came as such a shock when Chris Dana put a bullet through his brain. That's also why Dana's death transformed Montana into a national model for reintegrating combat vets back into civilian society.

3

Dana was a kid who joined the National Guard shortly after graduating from high school in Helena. Part of him died fighting in Iraq; the rest followed a few days after the Guard threw him out for having a bad attitude and failing to follow orders.

"That's happening all too often," said Steve Robinson, director of Veterans Affairs for the Veterans for America in Washington, DC. "Too many vets suffering from PTSD are being treated with disciplinary action. We need to be educating military commanders on PTSD."

War changed Dana. He wasn't always that way, his family told me.

"Before he left, he had a smile that could light up a room," said his stepmother, Linda Dana. "You were never quite sure whether he was laughing with you or at you. But when he came back, that light had gone out. He'd lost his essence."

"He was innocent," said his dad, Gary Dana, sitting outside on a porch that overlooked the trailer in which his son had lived. "He went to high school, played sports, and then he got thrown into the war. Growing up that fast was too much for him."

Chris was never an aggressive kid. He was one of the helpers. He was good with kids and liked them. His dad, who lives just outside of Helena and works construction, figured his son would become a social services worker and be happy helping people solve their problems.

Instead, Chris came home from high school during his senior year in 2002 and told his folks that a recruiter had visited their school and he'd signed up for the National Guard. That was a surprise, but it wasn't particularly alarming. America wasn't at war yet, and the discipline of serving in the military was considered to be a good way for teens to mature.

Right after high school, Dana went to Fort Knox, Kentucky, for boot camp and training, and then returned to Helena in 2003. He worked at a Target store and attended weekend drills. "During that time, he had no problem going to the drills, but after he got back from Iraq, it was an entirely different story," said his dad.

No one knows what happened

Chris went to Iraq with the 163rd Infantry Battalion, in what was the largest deployment of Montana soldiers since World War II. They were in the midst of some of the toughest fighting there was, but afterward, Chris couldn't talk about it.

"He'd tell us he'd been through a lot, then he'd drop it," recalls his stepmom Linda. "But then his eyes would just get vacant, and he wasn't there any more."

He could talk with his dad a little bit: "He told me that one time he was on top of his Humvee manning a 50mm machine gun when his sergeant yelled at him, grabbed him, and pulled him down. Had he not done so, a rocket would have decapitated him. And he said another time they took fire from some trees and returned the fire. Later, they inspected the site, but he said there wasn't much left of the guys."

He called home twice from Iraq, but spent much of that precious time talking about computer games and trivial things. "He kept things inside him because he didn't want people to worry about him," his dad said.

But a couple members of his unit told the Missoula (Montana) *Missoulian* newspaper that they were among the troops assigned to keep the first national polling places in Baqubah open, a tense situation given the fact that Baqubah sits on the edge of the Sunni Triangle and Sunni insurgents were determined to sabotage the election. After the election, their unit was ordered to provide security for the truck hauling ballots back to be counted. "The last polling place was a mile up the road, and we had a big concrete barrier to get out of the way," remembered Sgt. Dave Bauer. As they stopped to try to move it, an IED (improvised explosive device) blew up near them and rocket-propelled grenades (RPGs) showered down on them. "It knocked my commander out cold," Bauer told the newspaper. "I was shaking him, trying to wake him up, and another guy threw a pipe bomb at us from a bridge. We had the road unblocked, so we started going up it, trying to figure out who was firing at us."

They took the Bradley armored vehicle about three-quarters of a mile up the road to a grove of palm trees where the insurgents had retreated, and more RPGs were fired at them. One hit a power transformer, showering the soldiers with sparks and oil. Bauer grabbed the coaxial machine gun on the Bradley and opened fire, cutting the trees apart. Then an ammunition dump went up in a terrific fireball, and the squad cheered. "There were fires everywhere and trees were down," Sgt. Fred Hanson told the *Missoulian*. "There were Apache helicopters above us, but they didn't have to do anything. Dave took care of business."

Shortly after the 163rd returned in October 2005, Chris's company was disbanded and the soldiers were assigned to drill with other companies. Chris was ordered to drill in Butte, and it was a disappointment because it broke up a lot of close personal ties. He didn't see much sense in reporting for duty with a new unit, so he didn't. "Separating Chris from his friends was one of the worst things the government could have done," said his dad.

From the first day of his return, Chris was clearly struggling, clearly trying to put the best face on his problems so as not to worry his family, according to his stepbrother, Matt Kuntz. "The Christmas before last, he seemed to be doing pretty well externally. He was really proud and excited that he was returning home as a hero to his family. My sister and I asked him how he was. He said he was struggling, but he could handle it."

Bauer came back and was diagnosed with PTSD, and he knew what Dana was going through. "He was a young guy who would get into bed with his uniform and boots on, curl up in a fetal position, and fall asleep," Bauer told the *Missoulian*. "He'd never take that uniform off. He'd stay in it for weeks."

His family noticed other changes. He was real skittish, real jumpy. He didn't seem to like to be around people. "And he was real short with his dad," said Linda. "Gary would start a conversation, and Chris would shut him right down. I'd never seen him do that to his dad." And it got worse and worse. "He wouldn't take our phone calls," said his stepmom. "He'd go for five or six days of silence, then he'd call like nothing had happened."

Red flags for PTSD

To Matt Kuntz, a former Army officer and a Helena lawyer, the diagnosis of PTSD for Chris Dana seemed obvious. "You could look at his military personnel file and see PTSD," he said. "You could see a guy who'd been through a hard war, come home, and shut down."

Drugs and alcohol didn't seem to be a problem. Gary Dana is a recovering alcoholic, and he'd told his son about the dangers of abusing alcohol. He'd also told the boy that alcoholism runs in families and that his risk of abusing alcohol was higher than average. So Chris might go out on a bender with his friends occasionally, but it wasn't a regular thing. "He was a Pepsi guy," said his stepmom. "He wasn't much of a drinker."

They were able to keep an eye on him because Chris was living right across the road in a trailer that his dad had bought while Chris was in Iraq. He fixed it up, added an annex for a roommate, and invited Chris to move in after he got back. He charged a modest monthly rent of $200 apiece.

After a while, they noticed that Chris wasn't going to Butte for his drills and asked him about it. "He told us he was quitting, that he couldn't handle the drills anymore. Then I got an email that Chris wasn't reporting for his drills and asking me to look into it. And I got a call from Chris's Guard superiors. It wasn't 'What's happening to Chris?' It was telling me to get Chris there because he'd get a dishonorable discharge if he didn't go to drills," said his dad.

"I heard Gary take about three calls from the Guard, but they never asked about Chris, asked about his physical or mental health," said his stepmom.

"I could see that he didn't want to go back, that he didn't want any part of killing any more," his dad said. A childhood friend had moved into the trailer with Chris to keep him company, but could only watch his increasing isolation and depression.

Gary Dana tried to respect his son's privacy, not to interfere, not to get too emotionally sucked into his son's problems, although he did ask Kuntz, to see whether he could help Chris get out of the National Guard with an honorable discharge. "I told Chris what I'd done, and he said, 'Dad, why'd you do that? Why don't you just get out of my life?'"

Kuntz set up an appointment for counseling, but Chris cancelled at the last moment. Although it was getting harder to reach him by phone, he'd still talk a little. "During one call, he said he was really struggling, having a lot of trouble getting through his days," said his stepbrother. "I kept calling, but he quit returning my phone calls. I guess I called him for two weeks, but I finally figured if he didn't want me to help him, I couldn't help him. But I'm afraid now that I didn't realize how serious it was."

Planning his death

By Thanksgiving of 2006, Chris was avoiding his family even more. He told his dad that he'd have dinner with his mother, but he didn't. He just stayed home that day. "And he did the same at Christmas," says his dad. "He told us he didn't want any presents and he didn't want to do anything. So as a present, I gave him a month of free rent. That may have bought him one more month of life."

His dad didn't realize it at the time, but Chris was in the process of quitting his job at Target and spending his resources down. "In January and February [2007], he really started to spend money," his dad said. "I guess he figured when he ran out of money, it would all end."

In February, no one knows exactly when, Chris received notice of his less-than-honorable discharge, effective February 28. Typically, he told no one about it.

Kuntz was troubled and angered by his stepbrother's less-than-honorable discharge. "A lot of the people who have been our best soldiers and done our best work are getting real bad discharges," he said. "He quit going to his drills. He was so badly injured that he couldn't deal with the military any more." Kuntz wonders why the Army wasn't more sympathetic to Chris. "Instead of going out and seeing him in a non-threatening way, they made his life a living hell," he said.

Kuntz said his stepbrother's superiors in the National Guard called Chris to tell him that such a discharge would ruin his life by making him functionally unemployable. "Chris said, 'I can never stop working for

Target because if I do, I'll never get more work again.' Chris gave off every red flag. He was a good soldier who quit going to drill."

His roommate could also see danger flags. "His roommate said he was getting worried that last week," said his dad. "He was getting more and more quiet, and he wasn't working."

On March 1, Gary Dana didn't get the usual rent payment. Two days later, he figured he'd bring up the subject casually so he went over to his son's trailer with a couple of blankets. Chris's car was there, but at noon, there was no answer at the door. Late in the afternoon, he went back.

"Chris answered the door, and he looked groggy. He was pretty testy and I knew I had to watch what I said so I asked whether he'd been out all night and forgotten what day it was. He asked what day it was, and I told him the rent was due. He said he'd go into town and get some money. Then we talked some more, and I asked about his stepbrother, Matt, and his efforts to get his dishonorable discharge changed. He told me he'd told Matt not to bother. I asked why, and he told me it didn't matter. I started to ask why, but I knew he'd just snap at me, so I didn't say anything. I just told him I loved him, and he said he'd get some money and he'd call me in the morning."

That was Gary's last conversation with his son, and he knew something was terribly wrong. "I came home feeling awful, like something was happening that I didn't understand," he said.

The next morning, he made a point to be doing some yard work and wore his cell phone, but Chris didn't come out of the house and didn't call. At about 5 p.m., his dad called and got the answering machine. He was still close to the cell phone at 11 p.m. when the roommate, a nurse who worked nights and had just woken up, called to say that Chris had shot himself.

"The coroner says he probably shot himself about 5 or 6 o'clock," his dad said. "He put a .22 against his head and muffled it with a comforter. He said it probably made no more noise than a book dropping."

Gary Dana watched from his own home as the ambulance and medical examiner came and removed his son's body. Later, he went over to see if he could find any answers to his own questions. He found boxes of video games that Chris had bought, but never bothered to open. And he found a receipt for the shells dated February 27.

Congressional hearings demonstrate shortfall

U.S. Rep. Bob Filner, D-California, chairman of the House Committee on Veterans' Affairs, held a hearing recently that found the VA is not reaching the vets who need help.

"The VA mental health system is broken in function and understaffed in operation," testified Mike Bowman, father of Spec. Tim Bowman, who committed suicide in 2005. "There are many cases of soldiers coming to the VA for help and being turned away or misdiagnosed with post-traumatic stress disorder and then losing the battle with their demons. Those soldiers, as well as our son Timothy, can never be brought back. No one can change that fact. But you can change this system so this trend can be slowed dramatically or even stopped."

Noting a recent CBS television report that the rate of suicide among vets is double the national rate, Rep. Filner said, "The rate of veteran suicides has reached epidemic proportions. Suicide can be a very difficult public health crisis to gauge. I am more troubled by a lack of response by the VA than I am at not having perfect statistics. We need to hear from the VA what this agency needs in order to be able to reach out to all veterans. We know that the images of war trigger reactions in veterans from past conflicts. We need to go find Vietnam veterans and help them. We are not reaching the people who need help."

Half the VA facilities checked recently by the Inspector General's Office said they were attempting to identify at-risk patients through such methods as checking frequency of visits, utilization of outpatient treatment groups, and increased phone calls. But staff training was severely lacking. "Approximately 40 percent of all respondent facilities reported providing education programs for first-contact personnel that were mandatory; approximately one-third of all responding facilities reported inclusion of suicide response protocols; and a little less than one-fifth reported that programs inclusive of response protocols were mandatory," reported the VA's inspector general.

Further, it noted that the delay in receiving services was shameful. According to the inspector general, a vet seeking help for depression would receive an evaluation the same day at 40 percent of its facilities, 16 percent within a week, another 16 percent within two weeks, two to four weeks at 25 percent of the facilities, and four to eight weeks at the remaining facilities.

For substance abuse, 42 percent of the facilities gave a same-day evaluation, 24 percent within a week, 14 percent within two weeks, and 18 percent within two to four weeks.

A vet complaining of PTSD symptoms would get an evaluation the same day at 34 percent of the facilities, 17 percent within a week, 17 percent within a week or two, 26 percent within two to four weeks, with the remainder at a month or two.

And the inspector general said the VA should loosen its criteria for treating PTSD. Currently, only veterans with "sustained sobriety" get treatment, his report said.

An earlier trauma

Now Chris Dana's dad lives with guilt. "I keep wondering what would have happened if I hadn't gone over there to ask for the rent," he says.

Among the boxes, Gary Dana also found a small green notebook that his son carried during his year in Iraq. One entry from August 2004 was particularly poignant: "The last year I played baseball, we were undefeated. I turned 21 two days before I got deployed. When I was eight, my dad and me got into a four-wheeler accident, and he had been drinking. He quit after that. Went to Mexico spring break of my senior year."

Those disjointed memories of a life too short hit his father hard. "When I read it, I just broke up," he said. "How can you take a kid out of high school and make him kill people? What does that do to an innocent kid?"

Gary Dana has been sober for 15 years now, and his son's death was a real test. He said he badly wanted a drink to dull the pain, but he refused — in part because of the four-wheeler accident that Chris remembered. Chris was six, not eight, his dad said, and he'd been drinking most of the day before Chris got home from school. His son wanted to play, so they took the four-wheeler out joy riding. When they hit a gravel pit, the four-wheeler flipped. Gary managed to throw his son off the machine, but it came back and landed on Gary's head. His face was crushed. He lost his vision. Blood was everywhere, and he didn't know if he was going to survive. "We got the machine back on its wheels, and I told Chris to drive for help. I held on as he drove to a little store across the street. We must have had a close call crossing the street because I heard a car honk right beside me. When we got to the store, I was such a mess that one lady went outside to throw up. As a kid, Chris probably had some trauma from that accident."

Adding stress to stress

Previous trauma can make it harder for soldiers to deal with combat, agreed Dr. Rosa Merino, chief of psychiatry for the Veterans Affairs Healthcare Systems at nearby Fort Harrison, Montana.

Merino said preliminary data shows that about a third of the patients diagnosed with PTSD can begin to move on within the first year of treatment. "Another third experience symptoms for the next ten years or so, ebbing up and down," she said. "And the last group has been exposed to combat, but may have been exposed to trauma even before entering the service."

An estimated 10 percent of all Americans reportedly experience a form of PTSD as a result of repeated abuse, crime, or accidents.

In 2004, the Centers for Disease Control and Prevention tallied 32,439 known suicides, which made up 1.4 percent of overall deaths. That made it the 11th leading cause of death, with an overall rate of 11.1 suicides per 100,000 population. Among men between the ages of 20 and 65, that rate rises to about 20 suicides per 100,000.

But the VA can't provide comparable suicide statistics for its own vets. There are approximately 25 million veterans in America, with 5 million of them receiving health care though the Veterans Health Administration. Based on those rates, VHA mental health care professionals estimate 5,000 suicides among all vets, and 1,000 among those receiving VHA care. But those are only estimates, guesses.

An Army report, however, found that the suicide rate for its soldiers was the highest in 26 years, and that about a third of the 99 victims killed themselves in Iraq. It also said there was some evidence that the extended length of deployments could have been a factor in some of the suicides.

And a later Army study found that the number of military suicides was 20 percent higher in 2007 than it had been in 2006. Its 115 suicides was the highest number in more than two decades. And the number of soldiers who killed or injured themselves for some other reason was six times higher in 2006 than it had been four years earlier, 2,100 soldiers in 2006 compared to 350 in 2002. Part of that may have been due to a more sophisticated electronic tracking system, but clearly not all of it. Even though fewer than a third of those who committed suicide did so in military theatre, that was more than double the active-duty suicide rate before the terrorist attacks of September 11, 2001. During that year, the Army experienced a suicide rate of about 9.1 per 100,000 troops — by 2006, that had risen 90 percent to a rate of 17.5.

By early 2008, the Office of the Surgeon General was recommending improvements to the Army's suicide prevention plan. "Military suicide continues to be a significant problem in Iraq," it reported. While 10.5 soldiers per 100,000 took their own lives in 2004, the probable suicide rate for 2007 was more than twice that — 24 per 100,000. By comparison, the rate for the entire active-duty U.S. Army was 9.8 per 100,000 in 2001, but rose to 17.3 in 2006.

"People don't tend to commit suicide as a direct result of combat, but the frequent deployments strain relationships," said Col. Elspeth Ritchie, psychiatry consultant to the Army's surgeon general. And David Rudd, a former Army psychologist and chairman of the psychology department at the University of Texas, told the Washington *Post* that the increasing suicides raise "real questions about whether you can have an Army this size with multiple deployments."

Vets make up only 13 percent of the nation's population, but account for 20 percent of the suicides, according to the Iraq and Afghanistan Veterans of America. Male vets are more than twice as likely to commit suicide as men with no military service, and vets with PTSD are more than three times as likely to take their own lives as their civilian peers.

Among vets' groups, there's one dubious contention that surfaces from time to time. Some claim that more Vietnam vets took their own lives than actually died in combat. But to reach that number, you have to count: 1) every vet who died of a gunshot wound without leaving a suicide note; 2) every remotely suspicious accident; and 3) every fatal single-vehicle auto wreck. To my mind, that's unrealistic. Still the argument makes a good point — a true suicide rate must be higher because there are undoubtedly a number of vets who staged fatal car wrecks to take their own lives without losing insurance benefits for their families. And to add credence to that dubious contention, Thomas Insel, director of the National Institute of Mental Health in Bethesda, Maryland, recently predicted that, due to inadequate mental health care for vets, the number of suicides among Iraq and Afghan vets may ultimately *exceed* the number of combat fatalities.

Some vets file suit

A lawsuit filed against the VA by two vets groups, Veterans for Common Sense in Washington, DC, and Veterans United for Truth of Santa Barbara, California, contended that combat vets are about twice as likely to commit suicide.

"Troops who have served in Iraq and Afghanistan are killing themselves at higher percentages than has taken place in any other war where such figures have been tracked," it said. Pentagon statistics reveal that the suicide rate for U.S. troops who have served in Iraq is double what it was in peacetime. In early May 2007, a report was issued suggesting that 1,000 veterans under the care of the VA commit suicide every year. An additional 5,000 veterans who are outside the care of the VA commit suicide every year.

Another non-military study of 320,000 vets over the age of 18 found that male veterans are much more likely to take their own lives, often with a gun, than their civilian counterparts. "Male veterans are twice as likely as their civilian counterparts to die by suicide," said the study's lead author, Mark Kaplan, a community health professor at Portland State University who tracked subjects for 12 years. That finding is much higher than previous studies based on VA data. "Most veterans don't seek or receive care through the VA system, so we have to be careful about earlier studies," Kaplan said.

The VA Office of the Inspector General reported in May 2007 that the agency had to do a better job of tracking troubled vets.

"A comprehensive suicide prevention program must not only be able to identify those at risk for suicide, but ideally should identify periods of increased risk and should have a method for tracking at-risk patients to ensure that they receive timely and appropriate care," it said. "About 30 percent of the facility responders reported electronically tracking veterans at risk for suicide. Approximately one-fourth reported tracking veterans through the electronic medical record, while another five percent said that they were using other methods to track veterans."

Translated from government-speak, that means that 40 percent of VA facilities admit to not tracking suicidal veterans in any way, and two-thirds of them are merely giving lip service to the effort.

- 2 -
What are PTSD and TBI?

Behind the Faces of Combat are brains traumatized by what we now call post-traumatic stress disorder. There's a natural "fight-or-flight" reaction to the things that threaten us, but researchers are trying to figure out why some soldiers can't return to normal after the threat is over.

About 15 years ago, I was driving into town from my new home along the Missouri River just southwest of Great Falls when I noticed an old car with its turn blinker on, paused in the oncoming lane of traffic. I didn't think much of it until I was almost ready to pass it, and the car began edging into my lane of traffic. Going about 50 mph, I swerved onto the right shoulder, but the old car picked up speed and hit me right in the driver's-side door. That pushed me down into a ditch and up over a driveway, at which time my van became airborne. Somehow it also turned about 90 degrees and touched down sideways. When the tires hit the ground, the whole rig rolled. We were in the process of building a house at the time, and the rear of the van was filled with tile and paint samples that flew all over the back and shattered the windows. I remember seeing the windshield blow out in slow motion. When it finally came to a stop, mercifully on the rims of its tires, the door wouldn't open and I had to kick it out to be able to get out of the vehicle. Wearing a safety belt saved my life — I walked away uninjured, I thought.

I still drive that road today, and when I see a car stopped in the oncoming lane of traffic with its turn signal on, I get nervous. My mouth gets dry, my heart starts to thud, and my stomach knots up. I really want to stop, get out of my truck, and wave the oncoming car across the road in front of me. So one day I asked Eric Kettenring, the head counselor for the Vet Center in Missoula, whether these were signs of post-traumatic stress disorder.

"Post-traumatic stress," he replied, "but not a disorder yet. Remember that you weren't hurt, nor was anyone else. You weren't out in the field picking up body parts or trying to treat the wounded. And this only happened to you once. Soldiers in the field experience far worse things, and they happen two or three times a day, day after day, every day for a year or for 15 months. So you take what you feel and multiply it several thousand times and you'll begin to understand what PTSD feels like."

That gave me a much better appreciation for what I was beginning to see in returning combat vets. Technically, PTSD is defined as a series of persistent symptoms that follow exposure to a catastrophe or series of catastrophes that are outside a person's control and that cause feelings of intense fear, helplessness, or horror. For months or years, that trauma has the power to evoke feelings of panic, terror, dread, grief, guilt, despair, or depression. They may come back as persistent memories, traumatic nightmares, or psychotic re-enactments known as flashbacks, which are like watching a video without being able to turn it off. Combat vets usually find that flashbacks or intrusive memories are triggered by common sounds, smells, and sights. The sound of fireworks, the smell of diesel fuel, or the sight of a helicopter may trigger an involuntary rerun of a traumatic experience.

PTSD patients frequently find themselves emotionally numb in other situations or seek to avoid the situations that cause them pain. But by shutting down the negative emotions that lead to fear and panic, the emotional shutdown also blocks positive emotions, which can lead to isolation and divorce. People may be afraid to leave their homes because certain things may trigger symptoms. To be diagnosed with PTSD, they need to experience at least three of the following: emotional numbness, being dazed, losing contact with external reality, a feeling of loss of self or loss of identity, or an inability to remember parts of the trauma. These symptoms suggest a psychological state called *dissociation*.

And they frequently experience *hyperarousal*, which is like being constantly braced for the next barrage, unable to concentrate, unable to sleep. Anxiety levels are high, and some vets talk about panic attacks. Their emotional state significantly impairs normal functioning and normal relationships, leaving patients unable to help themselves.

"What is PTSD?" asked Dr. James Peake, secretary of Veterans Affairs. "You have to recognize that there are some normal reactions to combat. The things our men and women in uniform have to do will distress them, unless, of course, they are sociopaths. A lot of people returning from combat could benefit from some counseling to reintegrate with their families, but that doesn't mean they should be marked for life with PTSD. It just means they need counseling to help them adjust."

PTSD generally occurs after the threat has subsided, although prolonged exposure to combat can disable a vet in the field. The U.S. Army Office of the Surgeon General reported in early 2008 that "Nearly three times as many soldiers would be expected to report mental health problems at month 15 (of their first deployment) than would be expected to report problems at month one. Soldiers on multiple deployments report low morale, more mental health problems, and stress-related work problems. Soldiers on their third/fourth deployment are at particular risk of reporting mental health problems."

There are four different types of PTSD based on onset and duration. "Acute stress disorder" begins within four weeks of a trauma and lasts at least two days. Symptoms lasting more than four weeks are considered "acute PTSD," while those lasting more than three months are deemed "chronic PTSD." Symptoms that begin more than a month after the trauma are called "delayed onset PTSD." Combat, by its very nature, is a traumatic event, and greater exposure to combat frequently leads to more severe PTSD, complete with nightmares and flashbacks lasting for years, if not a lifetime.

Dr. Matthew Friedman, executive director of the VA's National Center for Post-Traumatic Stress Disorder, cited an Army study showing that rates of major depression, generalized anxiety, or PTSD increased from 9.3 percent before combat to as much as 17 percent for Iraqi vets, with the prevalence of PTSD increasing in a linear manner with the number of firefights a soldier had experienced. He said half the vets with PTSD are likely to recover within two years while another 20 to 30 percent will recover within five years. "We know that of women who have been raped, 90 percent will have PTSD symptoms almost immediately. By 12 months, that will be down to about 50 percent. Our data shows that 20 or 30 percent of them will never recover, but this data was developed before effective treatment was available, so it may be subject to change," he told me.

A look at the brain

To understand why combat vets like Chris Dana undergo so much post-traumatic stress disorder that they end up killing themselves, it's necessary to take a look at the brain and the damage caused by combat — the horror and guilt of killing another human being, the terror of having bullets coming at you, or having to experience the bloody aftermath. So here's a quick tutorial.

The brain is an astonishingly complex organ, which we currently can observe but don't yet understand. It weighs about three pounds and is 90 percent salt water. The main portion of the brain, about 85 percent of the total, is called the *cerebrum*. The top layer of the cerebrum, believed to be the last to evolve, is the *cortex*; the frontal lobe of the cortex, located directly behind the forehead, is the center for ethical decision-making, reasoning, planning, reading, and writing. The cortex is what distinguishes us from other animals and makes us human.

Below the cortex is the *mammalian brain*, also known as the limbic system, which governs pain and pleasure (fighting, fleeing, eating, and sex). It also appears to play a major role in the storage and retrieval of memories. Damage to two parts of the limbic system, the amygdala or the hippocampus, may cause recurring memories or a decrease in the ability to form new memories.

One of the major theories that neurobiologists are studying is that combat alters the relationship between the cortex and the amygdala. The cortex, our center of reason, receives the stimuli from our eyes and ears (although, interestingly enough, not smells — those go straight to the amygdala). The cortex then weighs the risk, measures it against past risks and other factors, and sends that signal to the amygdala, the brain's flight-or-fight center, and to the hippocampus. The theory is that combat overwhelms the cortex, which then fails to rein in the amygdala, which immediately goes into high gear figuring out how to respond to this threat. It also activates a portion of the brain called the hypothalamus, which can increase blood pressure, heart rate, sweating, and pupil dilation, as well as releasing a variety of hormones and peptides. Following combat, that imbalance continues, at least in part. That could allow the seat of emotional memory to become hyperactive, perhaps leading to nightmares and flashbacks.

It could also be dangerous because the neurochemicals involved in a heightened state of arousal can destroy brain cells. In the early 1990s, researchers found that stressed-out rats lost brain cells in their hippocampus, the memory center. A few years later, they found that combat vets with PTSD averaged eight percent less volume in their hippocampus than normal. Still later, they found an 18 percent reduction in hippocampus volume in patients who suffered from early childhood abuse and major depression. There have also been at least four studies showing decreased volume in the hippocampus of combat vets suffering from PTSD, which could explain some of the verbal memory deficits and perhaps some of the actual memory loss. However, other studies of twins — one exposed to trauma and the other not — suggest that smaller hippocampus volumes in both may demonstrate that size is a pre-existing vulnerability for the disorder rather than a consequence of it.

Brain cells are called *neurons*, and the human brain may have up to 100 billion of them, each enclosed in a very thin membrane that is capable of carrying nerve impulses. A fiber called an *axon* carries electrical impulses from one neuron to the next, while short branching fibers called dendrites receive those impulses. But an electrical impulse can't bridge even that tiny gap, so the impulse triggers the axon to release chemicals called *neurotransmitters* to stimulate the dendrite. Dopamine, serotonin, noradrenaline, and the opioids are a few of the most common neurotransmitters that deal with pleasure and pain. All of the brain's normal functions depend on neurotransmitters, and too much or too little of each can lead to serious disorders of thought, mood, and behavior.

Dopamine is normally the body's reward mechanism, rewarding us for doing the things that are good for our body. The high that a distance runner feels after completing a five-mile run is a jolt of dopamine rewarding him for exercising. In alcoholics, booze can commandeer the dopamine system and reward the drinker with a jolt of euphoria. And there's some evidence that excessive dopamine release may have a role in the hyperarousal and hypervigilance associated with PTSD.

In particular, there are a pair of oppositional neurotransmitters (amino acids) in our brains that co-exist in a delicate balance. Glutamate is the brain's primary excitatory neurotransmitter. It's quickly released in response to a threat, and it puts the brain into instant high gear. The opposite neurotransmitter is GABA, which slows the brain down during restful and non-stressful times, allowing it to filter out sensory information that's irrelevant. Each can override the other depending on the situation, but GABA is important because prolonged exposure to glutamate can damage or kill the brain cells around it. Some researchers are investigating the possibility that a shortage of GABA may be one explanation for PTSD and possibly even for depression.

Researchers have found one significant difference in the brains of those who may be predisposed to PTSD, the VA's Dr. Friedman told me. It's a difference in the serotonin transporter gene. Serotonin is a neurotransmitter that's been closely related to mood swings and anxiety attacks, as well as regulation of sleep and aggression. When an impulse leaves the axon, it triggers the release of serotonin. Some of it is picked up by the nearby dendrite, but some is left floating in the gap. The serotonin transporter gene is designed to recapture the leftover serotonin and pump it back into the cell for future use. And there's the difference.

Human beings can have a short form of the gene or a long form. The long form is believed to be more efficient in recapturing the serotonin. Since all humans have duplicate genes, it's possible to have two long genes or two short serotonin transporter genes.

"People with the double long gene are more resilient, while depression and suicidal behavior are more common among those with the double short gene," said Dr. Friedman. "And we've found the same to be true among people with PTSD. It's the first genetic difference, but there are many other probabilities."

Disorders such as PTSD, or mental illnesses, can be treated by medical doctors, psychiatrists who use various medications to restore the brain's normal chemical balance. In some cases, successful treatment can be done with a drug that increases or decreases the amount of a specific neurotransmitter, but most illnesses are more complex, involving several neurotransmitters at the same time. Doctors are still trying to figure out how to treat those illnesses, frequently on a trial-and-error basis for each specific patient.

What prevents a return to normal?

Such theories are persuasive, but Dr. Rachel Yehuda, one of the nation's top PTSD researchers at the VA's Bronx Medical Center in New York, wonders why the brain doesn't seem to recover after the threat is gone.

"The body is supposed to work that way," she said. "That rush of adrenaline helps you do what you need to do in response to a threat. For most of us, it's temporary. But PTSD is a disorder because something that should have been a temporary response is not. There's something wrong with the mechanism of getting back to the baseline normal."

Researchers at the Geisinger Center for Health Research found a correlation between combat veterans' use of both hands for common tasks and the likelihood of suffering PTSD. It found that soldiers who used only one hand for tasks — a measure of cerebral lateralization — were five times more likely to develop PTSD when exposed to combat. "These findings suggest the possibility of a pre-existing biological vulnerability for PTSD," said the study's principal investigator, Joseph

Boscarino. "We know generally what type of soldier is likely to suffer from PTSD before they get into combat."

While researchers look for a genetic explanation, Dr. Yehuda is convinced that the cause is both genetic and environmental. "Genetics alone cannot explain that vulnerability," she said. "It's not a slam-dunk certainty, but it's reasonable to suspect."

Early treatment may be one answer, Yehuda said. "Having these symptoms when you come back doesn't frighten me as much as having the symptoms of PTSD a few years after you come back. What we need to assure is that those symptoms don't turn into a permanent condition. There are treatments for PTSD. Particularly in the acute stage, early intervention may forestall a chronic condition."

New name for combat fatigue

PTSD has been around as long as men have been killing each other — and narrowly escaping death. Sometimes known as combat fatigue or being shell-shocked, it was a particular problem after the Civil War, in which countrymen split over the issue of slavery and slaughtered each other. Even during World War II, when America was defending itself against attack, it was a problem.

"I came back from World War II with PTSD," said retired Col. Bill Story, executive director of the First Special Service Force Association. "It took the form of extreme anger. I was very demanding — it was my way or no way. I dealt with those issues for many years through therapy."

Story's unit, the First Special Service Force, was the elite fighting unit that was the forefather of the Green Berets. It distinguished itself against the German Army in Italy, where Story remembers winning battles by slipping behind enemy lines and silently attacking enemy soldiers when and where they were not expected. "We were a group of young men trained to kill other young men in cold blood with a knife, or a garrote wire," he said. "We were simply trained killers."

PTSD rates soared after the war in Vietnam. One vet in three was estimated to have returned home with an emotional disorder, but that's only hindsight because PTSD wasn't adopted as a clinical disorder by the American Psychiatric Association until 1980.

Interestingly, that's about the same estimate that the RAND Corporation determined in the spring of 2008 for returning Iraqi/Afghan troops. In a voluminous 500-page report, it reviewed all the literature on PTSD, and did an independent survey of 1,965 service members and veterans, asking about PTSD and TBI; it also asked about major depression that could stem from a sense of loss following combat. "Unlike the physical wounds of war that maim or disfigure, these conditions remain invisible to other service members, to family members, and to society in general," it said. "All three conditions affect mood, thoughts, and behavior, yet these wounds often go unrecognized and unacknowledged."

Its survey found 14 percent screening positive for PTSD , 14 percent for major depression, and 19 percent for TBI. "About one-third of those previously deployed have at least one of these three conditions, and about five percent report symptoms of all three," it said. Based on 1.6 million soldiers serving in those two countries, it estimated that 300,000 would return with PTSD/depression and 320,000 with possible TBI. "As a group, the veterans returning from Afghanistan and Iraq are predominantly young, healthy, and productive members of society," it said. "However, about a third are currently affected by PTSD or depression or report exposure to a possible TBI while deployed."

Furthermore, the RAND report added, symptoms were more likely to occur months after the soldiers returned home, making the percentages in RAND's survey lower than what the eventual results might be. "The need for mental health care for service members deployed to Afghanistan and Iraq will increase over time, given the prevalence of information available to date and prior experience with Vietnam. Policymakers may therefore consider the figures presented in these studies to underestimate the burden that PTSD, depression, and TBI will have on the agencies that will be called upon to care for these service members now and in the near future," it cautioned.

Why so much PTSD?

Current rates of PTSD are already exceeding those estimated from the conflict in Vietnam, and there are probably five major differences between the current conflict and previous ones.

The *first* major reason for the staggering increases in PTSD, ironically, is the efficiency of our modern technology. In World Wars I and II, there were fewer than two soldiers wounded for each soldier killed. In Korea and Vietnam, that ratio increased slightly to a fewer than three soldiers wounded for each fatality. But in Iraq, 16 wounded soldiers are coming home for each casket. And by late 2007, the fatality count pushed past 3,800 soldiers, plus another 1,000 private military contractors.

SIGNATURE INJURIES

Civil War: Amputations from bone-shattering gunshot wounds.

World War I: Lung damage from toxic gases.

World War II: Radiation damage for those exposed to atomic bomb blasts in Japan.

Korean War: Circulation and joint problems resulting from intense cold.

Vietnam War: Illnesses from Agent Orange defoliant.

Persian Gulf War: Symptoms of the "Gulf War Syndrome," including fatigue, skin rashes, and shortness of breath.

Iraq/Afghanistan: Post-traumatic stress disorder (PTSD) and traumatic brain injury (TBI).

In 2003, the VA had projected that 23,553 soldiers would return from Iraq wounded and seeking medical care. Two years later, it upgraded that figure to 103,000. By early 2007, more than 200,000 vets from Iraq and Afghanistan have been treated at VA medical facilities, according to Linda Bilmes, a professor of public finance at the John F. Kennedy School of Government at Harvard University, and Joseph Stiglitz, a Columbia University professor who won the 2001 Nobel Prize for economics. More than a third of the soldiers have been diagnosed with mental health disorders, including post-traumatic stress disorder, acute depression, and substance abuse. Thousands more have crippling brain or spinal injuries.

Increasingly capable medical response teams are responsible for saving an increasing number of soldiers. Another reason is body armor and armored Humvees, which shield a lot of our young soldiers from death. But the body armor doesn't protect arms and legs, so the number of amputees has increased dramatically. And the explosions that no longer kill those kids bounce their brains against the inside of their skulls, a bone that's as hard on the inside as it is on the outside. That's why traumatic brain injury is becoming one of the signature injuries of this war.

To identify cases of TBI, doctors at the Walter Reed Medical Center in Washington, DC, screened all soldiers wounded in an Iraqi-Afghan explosion, along with those injured in a vehicle accident or a fall, as well as those wounded in the neck, face, or head. They found TBI in 80 percent of the cases.

Second, the rates from Vietnam were artificially low. We didn't know much about PTSD 40 years ago, and we didn't treat it aggressively. Soldiers coming home from an enormously unpopular war were called "baby-killers," and some of them were spat upon and shunned. They didn't want to call attention to themselves by seeking help. They wanted to hide. And it's only been in recent years, as they have become re-traumatized by newspaper headlines and televised fighting in Iraq, that many of them have been seeking help after four decades of solitary torment. In fact, therapists say that the upsurge in PTSD that's swamping them now is from re-traumatized Vietnam vets, not from Afghan and Iraqi vets. That tidal wave is yet to come.

Third, we have women in combat for the first time in a major conflict, and the rates of PTSD are higher for women than for men. Some of that may be due to a greater sensitivity among women. Some of it, however, may be due to a double whammy, with sexual abuse exacerbating the trauma of conflict.

Fourth, a greater burden than ever is being borne by our National Guard and Army Reserve units. Normally, these are weekend warriors, both guys and gals who feel good about drilling on weekends and helping with natural disasters like floods or forest fires. They joined the backup military forces without really expecting they'd ever have to go to war. But in 2005, half the fighting force in Iraq was Guard or Reserve forces. More than 210,000 of the National Guard's 330,000 soldiers have served in Iraq or Afghanistan, and the average length of their mobilization was 480 days. While the average age of the soldiers in Vietnam was 19, today's soldier averages 27 years old (33 years old for a member of the National Guard or Reserves). In addition, most Vietnam soldiers were single men; today 60 percent of those deployed have family obligations. Soldiers worrying about financial or family problems while they're deployed will have higher rates of PTSD. According to the military's Task Force on Mental Health, 49 percent of returning National Guard troops reported psychological symptoms upon their return, compared to 38 percent of active-duty soldiers.

"Our country never expected to use these troops as heavily as we have in Iraq and Afghanistan; consequently, after having been deployed, sometimes multiple times, these troops are experiencing rates of mental health problems 44 percent higher than their active-duty counterparts," concluded Veterans for America. "Based on available evidence, VFA believes that a considerable percentage of Guard members and Reservists have undiagnosed — and therefore untreated — service connected TBIs. Since our country did not expect to use these service members to the degree that we have, we do not have sufficient programs in place to treat them."

The *last* major difference has to do with length of service. Trauma builds cumulatively. The more fighting and the worse the fighting, the greater the likelihood of post-traumatic stress. In Vietnam, most soldiers were drafted for two years or volunteered for three, but they served only one tour of duty — and that tour was one year. In Iraq, more than half the troops have served two or three tours of duty, and more than 20,000 of them were prevented from leaving by the government's stop-loss policies, an involuntary three-month extension of deployment. The additional combat translates into additional stress, but just the uncertainty of not knowing when you will be allowed to leave adds an enormous amount of stress to an already overtaxed combatant. According to the military Mental Health Advisory Team's survey of soldiers and Marines in Iraq, soldiers deployed more than once were 50 percent more likely to have mental health injuries than those deployed just once. Since the beginning of the war, about 450,000 soldiers have been sent to war more than once.

Additional TBI only adds to the problem

Traumatic brain injury has been a concern for more than 15 years. In 1992, the VA designated four of its medical centers to provide dedicated beds and specialized staff to rehabilitate brain-damaged vets.

Scientists are also finding that traumatic brain injury is a lot more insidious than first thought, and it may take longer for this injury to manifest. Geoff Ling, an advanced-research scientist with the Pentagon, told *USA Today* that even though there are no outward signs of injury from a blast, cells deep within the brain can be altered and their metabolism changed, causing the cells to die.

The new findings are the result of recent blast experiments on animals, followed by microscopic examination of brain tissue. These experiments may mean that many soldiers, discharged but not diagnosed with TBI, begin to experience cellular death in the next few years. Symptoms can include memory deficits, headaches, vertigo, anxiety, and apathy, or lethargy. "These soldiers could have hidden injuries with long-term consequences," Ibolja Cernak, a scientist with the Johns Hopkins University Applied Physics Laboratory, told *USA Today*. Both researchers say the newly discovered cellular brain damage could be permanent, especially after repeated exposure to blasts, and lead to lasting neurological deterioration.

Early screenings at medical facilities suggested that 10 to 20 percent of the returning soldiers may have experienced head wounds, but it's hard to tell how many may have suffered brain injury. "We've had patients who've been in a blast who we tested. They looked OK. And they came back later and they were not OK," Maria Mouratidis, head of brain injury treatment at the National Naval Medical Center in Bethesda, Maryland, told that same newspaper. Apparently, the damage was so microscopic that it could not be detected with imaging tests.

"This is a new beast," agreed Alisa Gean, a San Francisco-based traumatic brain injury specialist.

At a recent conference on stress at CASA, the National Center for Addictions and Substance Abuse at Columbia University, doctors said they're still grappling with the increased prevalence of TBI. "We're finding that the diagnosis for TBI isn't very good because it is not reported very often," said Colleen A. Matter, staff psychologist at the Rochester, New York, VA Outpatient Clinic. "When a soldier is in a tank encounter with an IED that throws everyone around and the people are all bleeding, there's a good likelihood that everyone's brain has been bashed against the inside of his skull, which is just as hard as the outside, but they don't report that injury because they don't know they have it."

That's a standard line of questioning at the Minneapolis VA Medical Center, responded Dr. Paul Arbisi, associate professor and staff clinical psychologist. "We've been trained to ask vets how many times they've been involved in IED attacks. If they've been involved in 15 or 20 explosions, we know it's important to screen for TBI....

"We also know that if you're diagnosed with PTSD, you're 50 percent more likely to be diagnosed with substance abuse issues or depression," said Arbisi, who has a DOD contract to do post-discharge screening on Minnesota National Guard troops returning from Iraq. One of the things he'll be doing is looking at those who don't develop PTSD and trying to understand what prevented them from succumbing to it.

"Many [soldiers] report that their symptoms started after returning from combat, but others did not," he said, adding that DOD is interested in knowing why.

A more recent DOD study, reported in the *New England Journal of Medicine*, suggests that TBI may actually lead to PTSD. It said that one in six combat soldiers in Iraq may have suffered a concussion and that those injuries may increase their risk for PTSD.

In that study, conducted after soldiers had been home for three or four months, 2,525 soldiers from two Army infantry brigades (one active duty and the other Army National Guard) were asked to fill out questionnaires asking about missed workdays and dozens of other physical and emotional difficulties. The questionnaires also asked about concussions and their severity. The response was that 15 percent of the soldiers reported at least one concussion severe enough that one-third of them blacked out after the injury. About 44 percent of the soldiers who blacked out suffered PTSD symptoms, while 27 percent of the soldiers who reported less severe concussions also reported PTSD symptoms. Both are significantly higher than the 16 percent of soldiers the Army said will suffer PTSD symptoms without TBI. Those suffering even mild TBI were significantly more likely to report missed workdays, poor general health, medical visits, and a high number of other somatic and post-concussive symptoms.

"More than 40 percent of soldiers with injuries associated with loss of consciousness met the criteria for PTSD," said the study. "The data indicate that a history of mild traumatic brain injury in the combat environment, particularly in connection with a loss of consciousness, reflects exposure to a very intense traumatic event that threatens loss of life and very significantly increases the risk of PTSD."

Professor Richard A. Bryant at the School of Psychiatry, University of South Wales in Sydney, Australia, analyzed the study by writing that mild TBI can temporarily damage cognitive function and distort a person's ability to manage the consequences of psychological trauma, thus worsening the effects of post-traumatic stress. "There's a lot we don't know about these injuries, but we do know that context is important," the lead author of the study, Col. Charles D. Hoge, director of the psychiatry division of the Walter Reed Army Institute of Research, told the New York *Times*. "Being in combat, you're going to be in a physiologically heightened state already; now imagine that a blast knocks you unconscious — an extremely close call on your own life, and maybe your buddy went down. So you've got the trauma, and maybe the effect of the concussion is to make it worse."

Traumatic brain injury appears to be a long-term problem, according to the VA's Office of Inspector General. In a report released in early 2008, it tracked the progress of 52 patients who had been discharged from a VA hospital for TBI rehabilitation three years before. Three remained on active duty and eight showed no evidence of further VA care. However, the remaining 41 (79 percent of their sample) required ongoing medical assistance three years later.

"Specific attention to the long-term needs of those living with TBI is warranted, in part because cognitive and emotional impairments compromise patients' capacities to seek help on their own," said the study. "Unlike other types of injuries, brain injury often causes long-lasting emotional difficulties and behavioral problems. Further, in contrast to amputations and other disabilities, these problems are often not apparent to casual observers, even though they exact a huge toll on patients and their families."

To get a handle on TBI, the VA pledged to begin contacting nearly 570,000 recent combat vets to ensure they knew about medical benefits available to them.

Government has been underestimating the problem

Since the Iraq/Afghanistan war began, the Department of Defense has been struggling to understand the new realities of this combat. In 2005, the Army reported that 30 percent of its returning combat troops were reporting mental health problems within three to four months after returning from Iraq. In retrospect, that's almost certainly a low figure.

A 2006 study of nearly 8,000 returning vets by the coordinator for Mental Health Disaster Preparedness & Post Deployment Activities found a more serious problem: 57 percent of those vets could be diagnosed with PTSD; 45 percent could have depression; 32 percent had employment issues; and 25 percent had trouble with substance abuse.

Another DOD study of health care utilization in 2006 showed that among 222,620 Iraq veterans, 31 percent of them had at least one outpatient mental health counseling session within their first year back home.

"The challenges are enormous and the consequences of non-performance are significant," said the Report of the Department of Defense Task Force on Mental Health, June 2007. "Data from the Post-Deployment Health Reassessment, which is administered to service members 90 to 120 days after returning from deployment, indicate that 38 percent of soldiers and 31 percent of Marines report psychological symptoms. Among members of the National Guard, the figure rises to 49 percent. Further, psychological concerns are significantly higher among those with repeated deployments."

These studies don't seem to jibe with each other, much less with the Defense Department's independent review board, which put the number of vets returning with PTSD at about one in four.

"We're still trying to figure out those [PTSD prevalence] numbers," said Joe Underkofler, director of Veterans Affairs at Fort Harrison outside Helena, Montana. "Putting together the number being treated, the number resisting treatment, and the number with latent (undiagnosed) PTSD, I think a 30-40 percent figure is probably more realistic." Other mental health counselors suggest it will be closer to half.

The numbers also show a linear growth. As we look more closely at this problem, we're beginning to see it was worse than we had thought.

Situation only getting worse

But this problem is more than just percentages on a chart and more than just dollar signs. These soldiers are going to need medical assistance, many of them for a long time. And the VA is already overloaded. Vets seeking help face waiting lines of several weeks to several months, as well as an avalanche of paperwork that all too often is improperly filed or just lost. And some of the VA clinics don't provide treatment for mental health or substance abuse. Others require vets be sober before they can receive mental health treatment. And still others are already so overloaded that they can't accept new patients.

Things will only get worse because the bulk of our fighting force is still in uniform and still reporting to military doctors. We sent 1.6 million soldiers into Iraq and Afghanistan and 900,000 are still on active duty. When they hang up their uniforms, the VA estimates that its clinics may see an additional 750,000 new vets and half a million of them may begin visiting the nation's 200 walk-in neighborhood Vet Centers. And that doesn't include more than one million Guard and Reserve soldiers.

"One in three will come home with mental health issues, PTSD being the most prevalent," Paul Reickhoff, executive director/founder of Iraq and Afghanistan Veterans of America, told me when I visited with him in New York City. "The stats suggest 500,000 will end up with PTSD. Most of these people haven't even been discharged so far. And our system is already so overloaded that it can't keep up with the problem. So the number of vets coming home with PTSD is just going to blow this system. We're going to see divorce, joblessness, incarceration, and homeless vets."

It will be the aftermath of Vietnam all over again, Reickhoff fears.

And researchers are also finding that those suffering from PTSD tend to die younger. A study by Dr. Joseph Boscarino of the New York Academy of Medicine found that twice as many Vietnam-era vets diagnosed with PTSD died within 30 years of serving than did vets not suffering from PTSD. He found that the vets with PTSD not only had more emotional problems, but also suffered more physical disabilities, health problems, and medical conditions such as heart disease.

"This is the first study to confirm that PTSD is associated with a higher risk of death from multiple causes, particularly from cardiovascular diseases, cancer, and from external causes such as suicide or accidents," said Boscarino. "The reasons are unclear, but may be related to biological, physical, or behavioral factors associated with PTSD. We expected more deaths from cardiovascular disease, based on our past research, but the higher cancer mortality was a surprise."

- 3 -
A start toward reform

The suicide of former Spec. Chris Dana days after his less-than-honorable discharge spurred reform in Montana. For a year, the Montana National Guard looked at how it was helping combat vets return to civilian life... and what it needed to be doing better. Since Montana was meeting national standards at the time, America needs to do the same soul-searching because those standards aren't good enough.

Chris Dana's death stunned a fairly patriotic community and state. His stepbrother Matt Kuntz fired off a couple of stinging Op-Ed pieces to newspapers across Montana, and outraged letters to the editor began to show up in daily papers. More and more, citizens began telling state officials that it simply wasn't acceptable to treat vets like that. Gov. Brian Schweitzer quickly upgraded his discharge to honorable — "Talk about covering your ass," snorted his father — and directed National

Guard adjutant general Randy Mosley to appoint a task force to determine the severity of the problem and to find better ways of providing help to combat vets showing signs of PTSD.

As part of the process, the task force held a public hearing in Helena. A small but vocal crowd was present, accusing the National Guard of doing too little to help them after they returned from combat. "I may sound pretty damn angry and bitter, and I am," said Matt Kuntz, the stepbrother of Chris Dana. "We should have fixed this before. And the clock is ticking. If you think there aren't people out there right now staring at their guns, you're wrong."

Kuntz said the National Guard should have been able to identify the problems the vets are facing and have a program in place to fix them now, not a task force still trying to identify the problems. "Mandatory counseling for all vets is imperative while we still have them," he said. The National Guard's policy of asking soldiers to self-report their emotional difficulties through assessment forms mailed to them just doesn't work.

"The critical thing is to make some manner of counseling mandatory," he said. "There is no stigma that way. Since this is a self-isolating illness, you can't expect people to seek help."

Ken Rosenbaum of Helena, a helicopter pilot in Bosnia, was critical of what he called the Guard's failure to provide counseling for its members. "The Guard makes mistakes," he said, "and one of them is not identifying individuals who need help. That's a command failure."

Rosenbaum, also a Vietnam vet, said he's traumatized by watching the difficulties of his son, a 163rd Infantry soldier who spent a year working in some of the worst districts of Baghdad. "I want to scream," he said. "I talked to my son Sunday night, and there isn't a day that he doesn't think about committing suicide."

His son recently received treatment at a VA hospital in Sheridan, Wyoming, but he said it's important that all vets get the help they need immediately.

Vera Lynn Trangsrud of Shelby, Montana, agreed that counseling should be mandatory. "My son couldn't go to drills either," she said. "The night before, he'd break down, and his superiors who had not been to war did not understand why." Like Ken Rosenbaum, she said a day doesn't go by that her son, Michael Sheets, doesn't think about killing himself.

A call for help

That may be an overstatement, but not by much. Sheets, a former specialist E4 who was also a member of the 163rd Infantry, has been through a lot and has come close to killing himself on several occasions, he says.

Combat is all about death — preferably someone else's, not your own — and it takes its own toll. "Seeing three people blown into a million pieces is no fun," he said. Sheets logged about 250 combat missions during a year in Iraq and managed to escape unscathed as soldiers around him were killed or wounded. "We got called out to guard a mosque," he said. "One of our guys reached down for some water and got shot in the chest. I was watching people on the rooftops, so I didn't know it at the time."

But it came too close on September 21, 2005, the night his buddy, Travis Arndt, died. There were firefights all over Kirkuk that night, and Sheets was part of a quick reaction force, sitting atop a Humvee manning a 50mm machine gun. They rolled wherever the action was. "We were going down a road when we got hit by an IED [improvised explosive device or a homemade bomb]," he said. "Five insurgents jumped out and attacked us. They were well trained. They shot the top of the vehicle first (presumably to take out the machine gunner), then crisscrossed the rest of the vehicle with fire. They were all dressed in Iraqi police uniforms. We killed three of them and wounded another."

A little later, a car wouldn't stop and Sheets shot out its engine block. They arrested three Iraqis, all drunk, and found materials to make IEDs in the trunk. They turned the insurgents over to the Iraqi police, an exercise in futility because most of them were released within a couple of days. "There were a lot of IEDs going off that night," he said. "We were sent to a little alley where we were ambushed. We had fire coming from both sides. While we were getting out of there, we heard a radio call about an accident, a rollover. We knew it was bad because the lieutenant was kind of crying and said there was brain matter coming out of the gunner's ears."

Later, he heard that Travis Arndt had been killed just a few days before he was scheduled to rotate home on leave. Arndt had bought a ring for his girlfriend and was planning to propose to her, Sheets said.

"But it really didn't hit me much until I got home," he said. "Then I started getting nightmares and feeling guilty, feeling that I might have saved him if I'd hung back and shot back at them." Those nightmares brought back the terror of combat, night after night after night. "One nightmare that kept coming back was that my whole squad was getting hit, and I was screaming for help. My mom and stepdad came running downstairs to help. I didn't go to drill the next day, and the National Guard told me I was slacking — buck up and get a grip. They threatened me with a dishonorable discharge."

Alcohol seemed to help blur the nightmares, and Sheets began to close down the bars most nights. But even that didn't help much. "I kept getting nightmares about my squad getting all shot up. Usually I'd end up being the only one left, and I'd be trying to run and hide. It got so I really didn't want to go to sleep."

It got to the point that he wished he'd been killed in Iraq. "I felt I couldn't deal with it any more," Sheets said. "I came home one afternoon, walked past my mom and sister without saying anything, went downstairs, picked up my rifle, loaded it, looked at it, and then started to yell for my mom. She came running downstairs, and I just handed the gun to her. That's happened a couple of times."

Concerned, his parents made a doctor's appointment for their son in hopes that he could get some mental health care. The doctor recommended that Sheets see a psychiatrist, but it didn't turn out very well. "She told me it was impossible for me to be feeling what I was feeling, and I felt like she was calling me a liar," he said. He did demand and receive antidepressant medication, though, and is now working for a lumberyard in Billings.

"He was a lot more unstable a month ago," said his boss, Brad Partykia. "He would come to work and not talk to us. He was also drinking an awful lot. But that's changing since he got his meds. It's been a whole different deal for Mike."

His company commanders followed through on their threat and recommended a less-than-honorable discharge, but his recruiter got wind of the problem, went to bat for him, and managed to get him released with one that was honorable. "There are some decent people in the National Guard, but on the whole, they've treated me like shit," Sheets said. "I don't have much good to say about them anymore."

Low marks for mental health screening

Three months after Dana's suicide, the task force charged with assessing post-deployment policies concluded that Montana's National Guard has done a poor job of screening former combat vets for mental health problems.

"Painfully obvious is that the citizen-soldier, now a combat veteran, oftentimes needs services and support resources that extend far beyond what the Montana National Guard or the PDHRA program currently offer," said the Post-Deployment Health Reassessment Task Force.

It noted, however, that the state's National Guard put together its program "by the book" and currently offers more resources than required by the Department of Defense through the National Guard Bureau, the national authority for state Guard organizations.

"The Task Force considers the PDHRA program deficient," it concluded. "It does not provide the vision, operational conduct, or resources necessary to adequately identify medical or behavioral health issues that arise from deployment, or provide for proper follow-up and treatment either upon a Guardsman's return from deployment or in the aftermath when emotional or mental health issues often begin to emerge."

It specifically cited Chris Dana, his less-than-honorable discharge, and his suicide days later.

"The personal anguish that Specialist Dana endured is shared by many other combat veterans, their families, and their friends," said the task force. "It is our collective duty to recognize the inadequacies of the PDHRA program and thoughtfully identify and implement programs and processes that can truly serve those who served so honorably and selflessly on our behalf."

The task force came up with 10 problem areas.

The current system for assessing a vet's mental health during demobilization is "ineffective for identifying mental health issues," it said. Assessments often need to be more comprehensive and need to be performed in a confidential setting by professionals with adequate training.

"Veterans are hesitant to come forward with emotional or mental health issues," said the task force, citing concerns about negative impacts on their military and private careers, a perceived social stigma, and the personal pride of refusing to admit anything is wrong.

"If you need help, you're supposed to ask for help and it will be kept confidential," said Sgt. 1st Class Calvin James of the Montana National Guard's 163rd Infantry Battalion. "But it's *never* confidential. Everyone in the whole building knows before your supervisor does. Now most of our guys don't trust anyone and won't talk to anyone."

It said statewide availability of counseling resources is limited, particularly in rural areas.

"A specific centralized coordination and referral capability does not exist at the state or National Guard level," it said. In addition, veterans' organizations such as the American Legion or the VFW frequently have posts, but are not identified as a resource for Guard family programs.

The report echoed the concerns of Dana's family who said it was a poor idea to restructure the 163rd Infantry on its return home from Iraq, forcing soldiers to drill with new companies, because that isolated soldiers who had come to rely on their combat buddies. The report said such restructuring had "unintended and unanticipated consequences." Gary Dana noted that the restructuring was a national directive, prompted by the Bush administration's budget cuts to be able to spend more money fighting the war itself.

"Regulatory discharge processes and the nature of the discharges [less-than-honorable] for Guardsmen not attending drill periods do not take into account the affected person's emotional or mental health conditions," it concluded.

And it had 14 recommended solutions. The first was "Do not initiate discharge processes for an Operation Enduring Freedom (OEF) or Operation Iraqi Freedom (OIF) Guardsman for failure to perform (e.g., nonattendance at drill periods) until his or her physical or mental health status has been assessed."

The task force suggested creating a crisis team for at-risk Guardsmen. "The team's purpose would be to personally contact OEF/OIF veteran unit members who do not attend drill periods or whose wellness status is undetermined," it said. "The team will consist of, at minimum, a member from the Guardsman's combat team and a person with mental health training. The team is responsible for follow-up actions."

On returning home, Guard units have traditionally been given three months off to recover from combat trauma, but the task force suggested resuming drills immediately to keep the unit together as a support system.

"It looked good on paper, but we can't talk with our wives and kids about all that shit," said Calvin James.

Guardsmen with emotional problems should be referred to mental health personnel, and all Guardsmen should be enrolled in the VA health care system, it said. It also recommended a mental health assessment for Guardsmen within 90 days of returning home, then additional assessments every six months for two years.

"Expand the family readiness program to ensure that National Guard and Reserve unit families have access to support services at all times, including the pre-mobilization, mobilization, and post-mobilization time periods," the task force wrote.

Finally, it urged working with Montana's congressional delegation to expand the number of Vet Centers in the state and to provide additional funding "for its envisioned PDHRA program and for significantly enhanced family program staffing and services."

Montana's congressional delegation had already been briefed on the report and expressed its support, said Joe Foster, task force chairman and administrator of the Montana Veterans' Affairs Division. "That's important because some of these recommendations will need congressional support."

Adjutant general Mosley, who heads the state National Guard, has also embraced the report, he said. "General Mosley's response was to accept all the recommendations and plan to implement them. They have developed what they call a campaign plan that will address each of the recommendations and how the Guard will accomplish them."

Col. Jeff Ireland, director of manpower and personnel for the National Guard in Helena, said soldiers currently receive an assessment of the whole person, checking their physical and emotional health status. "We're proposing a campaign plan in line with what we received from the task force, expanding those reviews out to at least two years," said Ireland.

The Guard needs to improve its mental health resources, he agreed. "We don't have mental health professionals currently on staff at headquarters or at our medical detachment, so we're looking to bring some professionals on board," Ireland said.

He hopes to add two full-time mental health professionals at Fort Harrison, as well as four part-timers to join the medical detachments during weekend drills.

"We aren't currently funded for those positions, but General Mosley has taken that as an identified need to our National Guard Bureau and to our congressional delegation," said Ireland. "We're looking to increase our funding to bring those positions on."

When we are looking at solutions in chapter 16 of this book, we'll see how Montana has become a national model in assessing its soldiers for PTSD. But the National Guard has gone even further by hosting a series of community meetings across the state to discuss the emotional traumas caused by war with veterans of all eras, their families, friends, and caregivers. And as you will see in the chapters that follow, there's a tortured history of PTSD in warriors from Vietnam until now.

- 4 -
Women in combat

Some of the Faces of Combat are now female, and that presents some special problems. Nurses in Vietnam got PTSD just from caring for the wounded soldiers, but women are now carrying — and using — rifles in Iraq and Afghanistan. Further, they're finding there's the constant threat of being raped by fellow soldiers and officers, the very people they should be able to rely on for protection and support.

The war in Vietnam was universal, a pain shared across America, because the draft made it so. Forty years ago, virtually everyone had to serve. That's not the case today. Some of our soldiers are patriots who believe in the cause, but many of them are in uniform because military service is the best job they can get in a society where the rich are getting richer, while the poor are getting poorer. Military service offers decent pay, with medical, educational, and retirement benefits better than almost anything available in the private sector.

Today's Army is also different because it has opened its doors wider to women. Fifteen percent of today's soldiers are female. And they can serve in combat. Today, one soldier in 10 serving in Iraq is female. The 182,000 female soldiers serving in Iraq and Afghanistan dwarf the 7,500 primarily nurses who served in Vietnam or the 41,000 women deployed during the brief Gulf War.

"Our bodies aren't built like a male's, and we react differently, which hasn't really been in the newspapers," said Abbie Pickett, a former soldier with the Wisconsin National Guard. "No one's really dealt with how the female body is going to react to depleted uranium or a lot of things that are going on with male soldiers in high numbers."

And the treatment for women lags behind, as well. "There are some unique things we're seeing in women that we're not seeing in men," said Steve Robinson, a disabled Special Forces vet who heads Veterans for America in Washington, DC. "There are no programs across the board specifically for women. So they can't address issues like intimacy or fear for their families."

The poverty draft

Jamie Bender, a 38-year-old former Army combat photographer, is one of the women who thought the Army was a smart career move. "I was making six bucks an hour, but day care was kicking my ass. I couldn't make it. I couldn't make enough to get ahead," she says.

Born in Great Falls, she was a bright but angry child. "I was born a rebel. My mom got married when I was five, and I set out to make his life as miserable as I could."

School never interested her. "I knew homework was just a way of keeping me out of trouble, a way to keep me from doing the things I wanted to do, so I never did it."

By high school, she was a cheerleader, but ran with a rough crowd and skipped a lot of classes. "I partied a lot," she said. "I smoked pot and I drank, but no more than the people I hung out with. I got picked up for running away and being out after curfew, but I wasn't that bad of a kid."

In her senior year, she became pregnant and had to drop out of school. Bender's first child, Jeremy, was born when she was 17, and that load became heavier than she could handle.

She got a job as a store clerk, starting at $3.60, but working up to $6 an hour, and married a young man she'd met. "Our relationship was a struggle all the way. He didn't know how to be a husband, and I didn't know how to be a wife. I hated being a wife. He was very controlling, and I was very rebellious. If we hadn't been married, we wouldn't even have been friends."

A second child, Connor, didn't fix the marriage, and they divorced in 1992, Bender said. By this time, she was bouncing from job to job, but met an older man with a steady income and a nice home. They became engaged, but "at 22, he dumped me three months before we were to have been married."

She was bright, funny, popular, and the person that people turned to when they wanted advice about relationships and money. But she personally wasn't very good with either. "At the end of the year [1993], I found I was pregnant with Michaella and I still didn't have a place to live. I got kicked out of my mom's apartment. Then there was Mike and Jim and Doug. I was looking for love in all the wrong places. To be really honest, half my relationships were because I needed a place to stay. I was a walking ad for, 'Don't drop out of school.'"

A year later came the low point. Her overdue bills and rent took the remainder of her paycheck. "I had to put the last of the milk in my daughter's bottle and fill the rest with hot water. I had $5 for gas, but I didn't know the car needed oil and the engine froze. I had no money, no groceries, no car, nothing. I sat with my daughter on the side of the road and cried. That night, I gave a blowjob to a guy in a bar for $50," she said, her voice low and her eyes averted. "That night, I got the money to buy my child food."

Looking for a paycheck plus adventure

By comparison, the Army looked pretty good to Bender. "I knew it wouldn't be an easy time, but it was my chance to have a stable life with my family and with a steady paycheck and with all the perks that went with it. I knew if I didn't make it, I'd go back to making six bucks an hour."

A soldier just out of basic training makes about $7.75 an hour, but lives in a dorm and eats in a mess hall — so room and board is free. Married soldiers get housing allowances to compensate. There's full medical and dental care at no cost, and signing bonuses can go as high as $40,000.

She was looking for an adventure and a place to prove herself, but Iraq turned out to be more than she expected. She ended up in Ramadi, just northwest of Baghdad in September 2003. "At first, we were living in tents on a former Russian air base. There were 20 people to a tent, and the air conditioner didn't work — it was as hot as Satan's balls. We'd been there several days, and it was dark out. We were sitting around smoking cigarettes, and there was this big bang. The first sergeant immediately hit the floor, but I was just standing there, wondering what was happening. The next morning, a big 107mm shell went through four tents and hit a big piece of machinery … without exploding.

"We had a series of near misses," Bender said. "We had a shell that came through the PT [rec hall] and showered people with gravel. Our own shower tent was peppered with shrapnel. To this day, I can't go in a Porta-Potty."

Gunfire and bombs were constant, night and day. The explosions were a backdrop to everyday life, and Bender became resigned to never knowing whether she would live or die that day.

"The first few times I was in combat, it was no big deal because no one got hurt," she says. "Then I began seeing more dead soldiers, civilians, and kids. It became all too real, and all too senseless."

It also became more dangerous.

"A few weeks later, we were traveling from one base camp to another when three daisy-chained IEDs [improvised explosive devices] went off. Then we got RPG [rocket-propelled grenade] fire. I grabbed my weapon and my camera and followed the colonel. We chased them into a ravine and lost them. On the way back, we searched a couple of businesses. They were just a couple of garages with merchandise in them. There was an older Iraqi man and a couple of younger ones sitting in a circle with their hands behind their heads. Then I remember seeing this tall grass falling down, and I realized we were being shot at. Then everything stopped, and we turned the Iraqi civilians over to a rapid response team and went back to camp."

Adrenaline carried her through the shooting, but when it was over, Bender was overwhelmed. "It was so surreal that it didn't hit me until later that night," she said. "Then I started to shake. I took it personally — they were trying to kill me."

Sometimes that threat justified drastic measures. When Bender's convoy got hit by RPGs five or six times as it passed an abandoned building, they knew what needed to be done. "We just blew it up, took it away from them."

Bender's mind blocks some of that carnage. "I can't remember where we were going, but we got hit and a Marine in a different vehicle got half his face blown away. I don't remember much of that."

Although she was a photographer, Bender was also a soldier who carried — and used — a weapon.

"The first time I went out with the infantry, the first sergeant asked me if I would drop my camera if he ordered me to. And I told him, 'Hell, I'd throw it away if I had to.' I always felt that I didn't want my camera to get in the way of the battle. If my bullets would make a difference, I'd shoot first. I remember a visit to a school, and we got into a firefight. That was a major fight from which I didn't get many pictures. I shot my rifle instead of my camera that day."

Bender acknowledges that she had killed people, but said she's not ready to talk about that yet. Our interviews were short, no more than an hour. I stopped when I saw the stress shutting down her mind.

"For me, combat was always short and intense, but the aftermath was grueling," she said. "Even if I wasn't there for a battle, I'd have to take pictures of the damages. I shot [photographed] blown-up Humvees, blown-up soldiers, civilians, and children."

The bombs just didn't discriminate, she said. "Their IEDs were packed with shrapnel, and they would take out everything around them. There were people in those vehicles — old men, young men, women, and children. But we didn't kill them. We tried to save them."

Too much adventure

For Bender, everything changed on May 2, 2004.

"Our camp got hit," she said. "It was Sunday, and I was watching TV. It sounded like someone slammed a door, but I knew what it was — and it was so close. There were five Seabees standing around a Porta-Potty, and they got hit. One of them was blown back into the Porta-Potty. We lost one of our captains; he got some shrapnel in the neck. There were pools of blood everywhere. I took my camera down to the aid station and became invisible. My world shrank to what I could see through my viewfinder. I took pictures of chaplains holding hands with the wounded, medics working on victims, wounded soldiers being loaded onto helicopters.

"One image stands out in my mind," she said. "There was a soldier lying there in his underwear with a chaplain standing beside him. The soldier gave me a big thumbs-up. That's the first time I ever threw up in combat. We had five dead and around 100 wounded. And that's when I learned that there's no safe place in Iraq. I'd seen worse, but this was in my house. I wasn't outside the wire, out there in the war. There was no safe place for me anymore."

Suddenly, she knew it was no longer a choice between life and death. She knew she would die. "I went to see a chaplain and told him what I wanted at my memorial service. I wrote it all out."

Two weeks later, she was sent home and discharged with a 90 percent disability and a diagnosis of major depression and post-traumatic stress disorder. "But even today, I can't make long-range plans," she said. "I can't believe I'm going to live."

Echoes of war

Bender has trouble sleeping these days because she still hears the constant bombardment. "I still hear those sounds at night, and they're as real now as they were then. I really miss those moments when you're relaxing just before you go to sleep. Because that's when a bomb goes off for me. And that's what usually wakes me up, too."

And her nightmares frequently take Bender back to places she'd rather not remember.

Four of the seven soldiers she once played cards and ate chow with were killed when their convoy was hit by IEDs under a bridge, she said. "As we came up the road there were soldiers everywhere, gathering up the pieces of the soldiers who had died. On the side of the road was a little girl who'd gotten hit, too. The medics were working on her. She was the same age as my own daughter. That comes back to me three or four times a week. Sometimes in my nightmares, she becomes my daughter."

Bender photographed the memorial service for her friends, but remembers crying during it. Then her commanding officer came up and ordered her never to let her troops see her cry, telling her he'd have her sent home if she couldn't keep her emotions under control. "That's when I started building a wall around my feelings, compartmentalizing my emotions," she said. "And when I came home, I didn't feel anything at all. It was like living with strangers. It took a year before I started feeling feelings again."

Within an hour of that memorial service, four more friends died in another convoy and Bender was once again dispatched to the scene with her camera. In addition to the American soldiers, an Iraqi man died when his old pickup truck was hit and became engulfed in flames. Her colonel really wanted pictures to demonstrate that the Iraqi insurgents were killing their own people. "The body was all black," she said. "The skin on his skull was flaking off, and you could see the bone. I had to make sure I photographed him from every angle."

The carnage was constant. Frequently, she was afraid to look away from her camera viewfinder. "Once in the road, I saw a hand in a fingerless glove," she said. "I remember thinking to myself that this guy might be a mechanic because his nails were so dirty." Another time, she found herself standing beside a shredded vest with a spinal cord enmeshed in it. At another blast, she encountered a boot split open with toes sticking out of it. "Mortuary affairs guys brought out their body bags and began filling them up, and I remember wondering how they know who goes with who."

Those scenes now torment her nights. "When I have dreams about body parts, I'm never sure whether my dreams are real because it seems so real — everything that I'm seeing or feeling or hearing seems real to me. But other dreams are more surreal; there's no color or sound. My worst dream is seeing that black body again, only I know it's my son. It opens its eyes, and it's my son's eyes."

Sexual assault, a double whammy

"And then there's the night I was raped," says Bender, struggling to keep her voice level. It's a topic she's been avoiding over weeks of interviews with me, so volunteering it takes incredible courage. Her therapist, Christine Krupar, has joined us to help her through this session.

The rapists were apparently two of her fellow soldiers at a forward operating base she had been visiting that day. "It was pitch black, and I was walking alone," she said. "I shouldn't have been walking alone."

Two men pulled her into the bushes, ripped her uniform off, and raped her, she said. "I remember thinking to myself, 'I hope this isn't really happening because I don't think I can handle this.'" After it was over and they had left, she put her clothing on and stumbled back to her room. "I was all dirty. I washed myself and my clothes, and I tried not to think about it. I didn't sleep that night, but I reported for work the next morning. And I never reported it. But it taught me a lesson. I never turn my back on anyone. I never trust anyone, even if I think I can."

That's all too common, said Krupar, a former police officer turned counselor who has been specializing in PTSD cases, including Bender's. "Since I've been working with vets, I keep hearing stories of rapes and murders and brutal beating and other atrocities," she said. "I keep hearing of terrible things they've done or watched done without doing anything to stop it."

That's the nature of war, responds Bender. "We just get hard. We stop caring about women and kids."

But it seems to go beyond that. In war zones there's nothing to prevent unabashed power; the rule of law no longer applies. "Some soldiers really believe they can do anything they want," said Bender. "They say, 'If you don't like what I'm doing, I'll shoot you.'"

Greater emotional carnage

Experts are finding that female soldiers are experiencing higher rates of PTSD than their male counterparts, and some of that may be a result of sex abuse. A VA study of 60,000 soldiers with PTSD found that 22 percent of the women suffered from MST, military sexual trauma, which includes sexual assault and harassment. And that's probably a low figure, since counselors say many women have trouble reporting MST due to a fear of retaliation by their superior officers.

An analysis of several hundred studies reported in the American Psychological Association's *Psychological Bulletin* suggested women are twice as vulnerable to PTSD as men. In general, it found that women were more likely than men to develop PTSD when both underwent the same experiences. Other studies have shown that men are more likely to have experienced more severe trauma over their lifetimes, but women are more likely to be affected by the stressors they're subjected to.

In the Vietnam era, PTSD rates for female soldiers were about four percentage points lower than for males, but that may have been because sample sizes were much smaller and women were generally assigned to roles as nurses. After the Gulf War, however, Army data showed 16 percent of the women met the diagnostic criteria for PTSD, twice the rate of the males, despite the fact that their combat exposure was relatively low. The larger sample size for the latter figures gives it greater credibility.

One factor may be that little girls are subjected to greater trauma, including molestation and childhood assault. A study in the Detroit area showed that 13 percent of the women showed signs of PTSD, compared with 6.2 percent of the men. It may be that women experience more traumatic events, such as being choked, beaten, threatened with a gun, or raped by an intimate partner or family member.

But military sexual assault is also suspected to be one of the main causes for PTSD. It's not that our female soldiers are being raped by the enemy. Some of them, however, have been raped by their fellow soldiers. And many more of them have been pressured into sexual relationships with their sergeants, according to Sara Corbett, writing for the New York *Times*. She said those relationships have become so common they're referred to as "command rape."

A 2003 VA study found that nearly one-third of a national sampling of female soldiers seeking health care reported that they experienced rape or attempted rape during their time in the service. Of that group, 37 percent of them said they were raped multiple times, and 14 percent of them reported gang rape. Some studies have shown the sexual trauma to be *more stressful* than combat trauma, but the combination provides a significant double whammy.

It seems unthinkable, outrageous, that female soldiers would fear being raped by their colleagues. But remember that these soldiers are a world away from civilized society and its moral values or laws. They're struggling in foreign countries that they don't understand, fearing death at any moment, getting little sleep, and sweating in full battle gear with temperatures well over 100 degrees. It must seem like a nightmare.

Remember also that many of the victims are women like Bender, women who had previously struggled in a civilian world to make it any way they could. Many of them will come into military service bringing a load of emotional baggage with them, only to add a layer of combat stress on top of it.

Officer rape is not consensual

Sexual assault is also at the root of Abbie Pickett's problems. Ever since the 24-year-old combat-support specialist with the Wisconsin Army National Guard was raped by a drunken officer walking her back to her base after a party, she has rebelled against military authority. "I had a chip on my shoulder, but I didn't realize it," she told me, sitting in a coffee shop near the Edgewood College campus in Madison, Wisconsin. "Even without being in combat, I think I would have come home with PTSD."

But a triple-whammy mortar attack on her base in Iraq made that probability into a certainty, she added.

Pickett joined the Wisconsin National Guard at 17 with her parents' reluctant permission. Not long after she'd gotten out of basic training, her unit was sent on a humanitarian aid mission to Nicaragua. Seeing the kids in poverty and being able to help was a wonderful feeling, she said. But that changed the evening everyone was relaxing at a hard-drinking booze bash in their camp. "I was drinking with a bunch of officers, and I was fairly drunk. One guy and his buddy said they'd walk me back to my camp and I knew this wasn't going the right way, but I was only 19 and I didn't know how to handle it. I remember running into a Marine I knew and asking him to walk me home, but he backed out."

Instead, the officers walked Pickett into the woods where one sexually assaulted her while the other stood guard. She didn't fight it, she said, because she felt powerless. And she didn't report it for the same reason: it was a superior officer. "It was a sexual assault by someone with more power and rank," she said.

Diane Castillo, director of the VA Medical Center in Albuquerque, New Mexico, told the Albuquerque *Tribune* that of the 188 women being treated for PTSD in her clinic, between 80 and 90 percent of them reported some sort of sexual trauma while in the military. That trauma can range from rape to harassment, she said.

"Imagine being out there in a war zone, worrying about the enemy, and then also having to worry about being raped by your own comrades," said Castillo. "It's a double stressor, and there's nowhere to turn."

Castillo said some female vets told her that they took a gun with them on trips to the latrine because they worried about sexual assaults. Others never visited the latrines at night, and still others said they never went alone.

The military remains a sexist outfit, she concluded. "In the military culture, women are pushed into one of two roles — either you date men and you're a whore, or you don't and you're a dyke. That's true to some extent of society as a whole, but it's much more true of the military."

For many female soldiers, reporting such assaults seems pointless because the men deny it, and their higher rank gives them greater protection and credence. Department of Defense statistics bear out the futility. Investigations into 3,038 sexual assault complaints in 2004-05 showed that more than half were dismissed out of hand, roughly 20 percent were resolved through administrative punishments like demotions or transfers or letters of reprimand, while only 329 of them — about 11 percent — resulted in the court-martial of a perpetrator.

When her unit returned home, Pickett tried to forget the incident, but couldn't. "I came home and changed my life, dropped my boyfriend, switched jobs, bought a car, and just tried to forget it ever happened. I tried dating a little bit, but it didn't stick. I don't know why, but I wasn't connecting all the dots."

War within a war

Being vulnerable makes people more sensitive to other injustices, and a sharp mind and a quick tongue kept Pickett at loggerheads with her commanders. That only got worse when the Wisconsin National Guard was sent to Iraq in May of 2003. Her job was to drive a refueling truck filled with 2,500 gallons of diesel fuel for more than 140 pieces of equipment, stuff like generators, dump trucks, loaders, scrapers, and haulers — all the equipment needed to build roads or checkpoints. But she kept getting furious with the stupid orders her officers would hand down. "Every day, there would be the senselessness of people imposing their authority on you just to display their power," she said. "And as a sexual assault victim who had her power stripped away from her, I felt it more keenly."

She remembers an officer who decided that the soldiers were paying too much attention to all the dogs hanging around camp looking for a handout. He ordered them all shot, and Pickett was outraged at the senseless slaughter. Another incident involved a work detail on a Sunday when she wanted to attend a church service in the morning and then join a convoy in Tikrit where she could use a telephone to call home. She asked to have the work detail delayed to another day, but her request was denied. She remembers asking, "Sir, are you forcing me to choose between my God and my Mom?" And she remembers the response: "Pickett! In my office! Now!"

And the pornography was a particular problem for a rape victim. "There were boxes and boxes of pornography, and the guys were watching it all the time," she said. "You'd walk into a room, and the pornography was on. It was everywhere, and no one even tried to hide it. It was out in the open, everywhere."

She remembers being depressed and then feeling suicidal, so she said she visited the camp medic and was prescribed antidepressants that made her feel a little better. "Even without the combat situations, I would have come home with PTSD," she repeated. "It was always an uphill fight. The war within the base *was worse* than the war outside it."

War comes home

Well, almost. That changed when the war outside the base at Baqubah, just north of Baghdad, came inside it.

Pickett had just left the chow hall after supper and had gone to the rec hall to hang out for a while. She dropped her Kevlar helmet and flak jacket near the door, then checked the guys playing ping-pong to see if any of her friends were there. As she watched, she heard the familiar thud of a mortar. That thud usually is the distant sound of its impact and explosion, but a good soldier is always alert for a couple of seconds to assess the possibility that the first thud might be the launch of a nearby mortar, which could be a real danger. Since mortars often come in clusters of three, one near miss could be followed by death.

"The next thud shook my body and made it clear that we were under fire," said Pickett. "One of the big guys hit the ground, and I ran outside and crouched beside a wall. I could hear another mortar coming in, and there was a huge explosion. The next thing I heard was a scream. A girl was screaming, 'The bone is coming out of my arm!' I ran over and felt her arm, and it felt OK, but she just kept screaming. I wanted to punch her to get her to shut up. Then someone called for a medic inside, so I ran inside. There were four bodies on the floor. I asked who was hurt the worst, and a guy nodded toward the girl next to him and said, 'She is.'"

As Pickett began to use her first aid training on the female soldier, she noticed that blood covered the floor, but the girl didn't appear to be bleeding that badly. "So I said to the guy, 'Is this all hers?' and he said, 'No, I got hit, too.' I lifted up his arm and the artery was hit — it had been taken out by a piece of shrapnel — and the blood just started squirting all over."

Then the first of the medics hit the scene and began emergency triage, so Pickett ran for a truck. "I ended up transporting five patients —

the four from inside and the one outside — to the hospital in blackout conditions. When we got there, my pants and boots were covered with blood. As we unloaded them, more patients kept coming in from the chow hall, where another mortar had hit. And then a mortar hit the hospital. We immediately covered our patients with our own bodies, but it didn't detonate and no more came."

As she thought about it, Pickett grew more and more furious. "Obviously, someone knew our base very well. They hit the chow hall and the MWR [rec hall], then waited and hit the hospital about the time they figured the victims would be getting there. And that made me really angry. I had tried to be humanitarian in Iraq, to help people, but I began to wonder whether the people we were feeding during the day were bombing us at night. That made me really angry, and I wanted to go out on missions and blast people and kill them."

It also forced her to accept her own death. "When you're in the kill zone of a mortar, you're supposed to die. So I figured I might as well go ahead and get it over with."

Hell at home

When Pickett returned home, the mental health assessment tests clearly showed danger signs. "I'd been on antidepressants and sleeping pills in country, and I'd seen a lot of dead or injured Iraqis and Americans. The mental health ops gave me a 30-day supply of antidepressants and a toll-free number to call to get counseling in Wisconsin. The first two numbers I called had been disconnected, and the third was in Madison … New Jersey. I was talking with them about where I was and where to go for counseling, and it just didn't make any sense. Finally, we figured out that they were in New Jersey and I was in Wisconsin. So I called the toll-free number again, and they gave me the same three phone numbers."

Her depression grew, and she kept thinking of killing herself. "For the first few months after I returned, I only slept in 50-minute increments, walking up repeatedly through the night," Pickett said. "And I've never slept well since."

As her antidepressant supply dwindled, she got desperate and called nearby Camp McCoy to demand help. Finally, she showed up and was given another 90-day supply.

"I never had any trouble seeing regular VA doctors, and they'd make a call to the mental health doctors to say I was in the office and feeling suicidal, but I never really got any help," she said. "I saw a mental health counselor for about three months, missed an appointment, tried to reschedule it, and for the next seven months the ball was completely dropped."

Pickett was trying to go to college, and she found herself dropping from an honor roll student to someone barely able to hang onto four credits. "I was having a hard time getting out of bed during the day. The radiators in my house would make a high-pitched whine that sounded just like an incoming mortar, and they were really freaking me out until I learned how to turn them off. I was getting no help from anyone, and I couldn't help myself. When you can't comb your hair or brush your teeth because it takes too much out of you, you certainly can't get on the phone and fight with the VA to demand help."

About a year after her return from Iraq, Pickett was finally awarded her VA disability, a 70 percent disability rating due to PTSD. A private therapist realized that her antidepressants were making her feel worse and changed her meds for the better. She got involved with the Iraq and Afghanistan Veterans of America and began to find her voice, healing herself by helping other disabled combat vets.

She remembers running into Wisconsin Lt. Gov. Barbara Lawton, who asked how things were over there. "I told her that to be quite frank, the war within the gate was much worse than the war outside it. She said, 'Come into my office right away.' I told her about the leadership problems, what I experienced, and even problems with the VA. And she really started to help out. She called the National Guard leadership on the carpet. And she was the first to help me understand that pornography is not OK."

Pornography is an issue she's finally coming to terms with. "I had accepted the fact that guys would be guys, but I'm beginning to understand that it's not OK. I guess I thought that when guys are away from home and away from sex, it's better than raping someone. But it's not right to degrade women, and maybe it leads to more problems."

Pickett's nightmares are still frequent and intense. "Many of them are about that moment right before you die. Sometimes I also get the mortar attack, but it's all about being helpless and there's nothing you can do."

But she's learned to yell out in her sleep and wake up her boyfriend for help. Just being able to experience intimacy again is a step forward for Pickett, a slender and articulate blonde now working on her bachelor's degree in political science and psychology at Edgewood College.

"Things have really changed since Chris entered my life," she said. "Sometimes I wonder what it's like for him, but he seems to take it pretty well. Sometimes I just cry and he doesn't know what's wrong. It's pretty hard for him."

Specialized help for women

Recently, a handful of VA programs have sprung up around the country offering 60- or 90-day treatments specifically for women. And the women who are seeking help have been through some severe combat, Darrah Westrup told *USA Today*. "Women are talking about dismembered bodies, seeing their buddies blown up in front of them," said Westrup, who manages a women's program in Menlo Park, California. "They're trying to reconcile, 'I have killed people.'"

Although women are barred from ground jobs in infantry, armor, and artillery units, there's no safe place in Iraq or Afghanistan. And some of the support jobs to which women are assigned are just as dangerous as any other. The risk is equally high for women driving supply convoys or guarding checkpoints or searching women during neighborhood patrol operations. According to the Pentagon, more than 100 female service members have been killed and 570 wounded in Iraq and Afghanistan.

The disability toll for emotional trauma is far worse. In 2006, nearly 3,800 women diagnosed with PTSD were treated by the VA, accounting for about 14 percent of all vets treated for PTSD that year. And yet, that's almost certainly an understated figure.

The Defense Department's Mental Health Task Force reported that many female combat vets needed treatment, but refused to seek it due to "their need to show the emotional strength expected of military members." It also said that many female vets didn't view themselves as vets and didn't realize they were entitled to the help they needed and deserved.

In addition, the VA said that 20 percent of the women it has treated since 2002 showed symptoms of military sexual trauma. For military women, sexual abuse by their fellow soldiers is "an unnecessary betrayal," Westrup told *USA Today*. "Most go over understanding the nature of war."

Special emotional issues

Female vets need special attention. Some recent-era vets have served in combat, but others who served in earlier combats need an equal amount of attention. Some of those served as nurses and witnessed firsthand the pain and futility of being unable to save the soldiers in their care. Many still deny their pain because they don't feel justified when others went through a more direct trauma. They may also deny a misdirected guilt over soldiers' deaths. Some may still be haunted by the intrusive faces of those who died in their care. Remember that these caregivers are the most sensitive to PTSD because they went into combat with such good intentions.

One of the most effective treatments is to point out the thoughts they deny. They should know that their distress is no less severe than combat vets. And they should be reminded of their achievements in providing comfort to soldiers who would otherwise have died alone.

All of them have actions they can be proud of, and they need to be reminded to give themselves credit for those things, said Diane Carlson Evans, a former Vietnam War nurse from Helena who founded the Vietnam Women's Memorial Foundation in Washington, DC.

"After Vietnam, there was a lot of quiet suffering that would only come out years later," she told me. "Studies have shown that women have not gone for help for many years, suffering in silence because they feared reporting their problem. One thing we learned from Vietnam is that women have no place to go. If we're assaulted or raped, we could go to our commanding officer, but we may not be believed. The victim, as the accuser, may be moved to a different post, transferred out, or not get a promotion in cases where she was assaulted by a superior officer."

Women in the military have a legitimate fear of being captured by enemy forces, assaulted, and raped. "But it's worse in a war zone, where you have to worry about the enemy, our own military counterparts, or our own forces. MST [military sexual trauma] is fairly high. One woman who was a trauma nurse told me she's afraid to go to the bathroom at night because women walking to the latrines alone were attacked and assaulted. Now there's not only the fear of everything that goes on in a war zone, but also the fear of being assaulted," she noted.

Adding to the danger is that everyone is armed: the enemy, other soldiers, and the women. "We're human beings, and our morality is 'should we really be shooting these people?'" Carlson asked. "Men traditionally go off to war trained to shoot the enemy. They do what they're asked to do. But women in general get great angst in taking lives. I know that, as a mother, I certainly do."

Carlson served one tour in Vietnam in 1966, then worked with wounded soldiers in military hospitals through 1972. A decade later, she began to realize that she was suffering the effects of PTSD. When she sought help at the VA hospital in Minneapolis in 1983, they told her she was the first female vet they'd treated there. "In Vietnam, we were shot at, but we could not shoot back. That's a major difference from the women coming back from Iraq today. I guess the other difference is that we were not out on patrol, but the women today are. And women and men are mingled, which contributes to a great deal of stress. We're seeing so much MST today that the VA may have to open new units just to treat it."

In looking at the damage that we're doing to these young women, I have to conclude that it was a poor decision to allow them to go into combat. Emotionally, women are caregivers. They are designed to raise children and to keep them safe. I think we need to pull the women off the battlefields and away from the soldiers who may try to take advantage of them. Simply caring for the wounded can be traumatic enough for women, as a whole generation of Vietnam nurses can attest to.

Photographs
by Jamie Bender

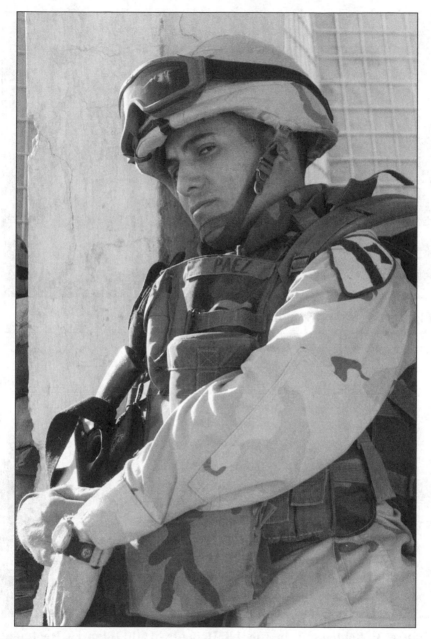

Figure 1: On duty.

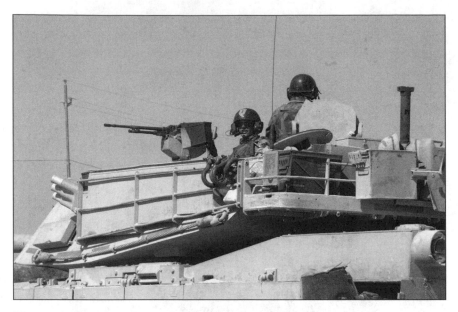

Figure 2: Constantly on the lookout for attacks.

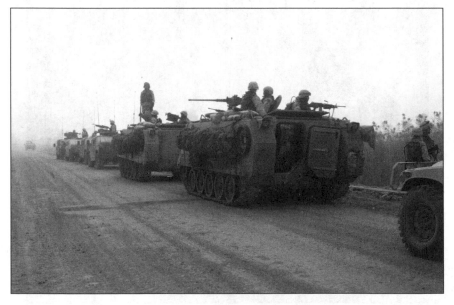

Figure 3: Soldiers from the 1st Brigade, 16th Infantry Regiment pause on a road outside of Ramadi.

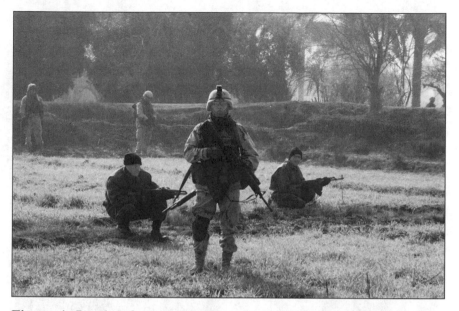

Figure 4: Iraqi defense soldiers are trained to patrol by American infantry soldiers.

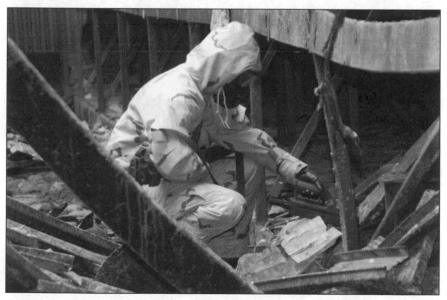

Figure 5: A soldier in protective chem gear checks a possible chemical weapons site. Nothing was found.

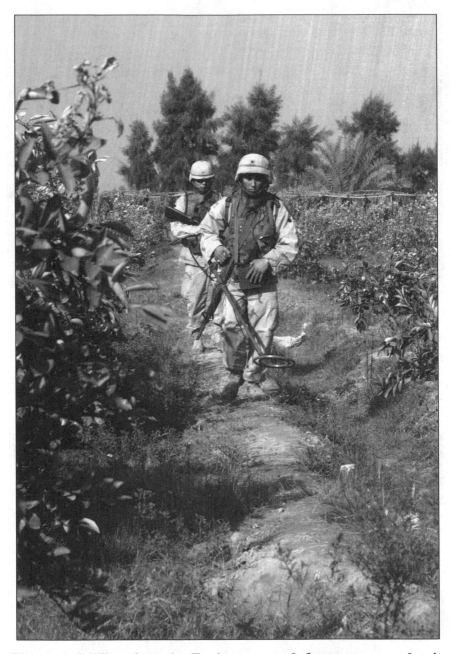

Figure 6: Soldiers from 1st Engineers search for weapons caches in an orange grove.

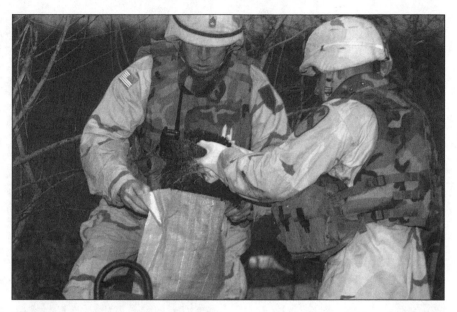

Figure 7: A soldier's remains are recovered and placed in a sandbag for transport to mortuary affairs.

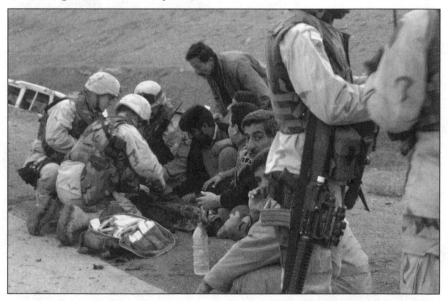

Figure 8: Medics work on a young Iraqi girl injured in a vehicle-borne IED explosion. Three soldiers and the girl died in the attack.

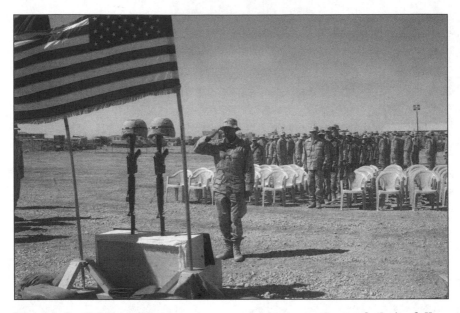

Figure 9: Soldiers line up to pay respects to two of their fallen brothers.

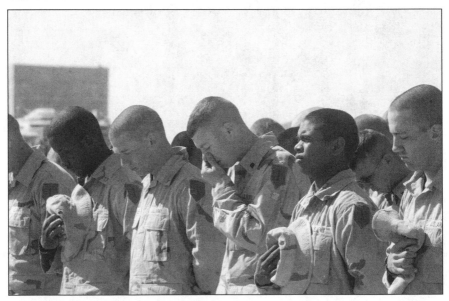

Figure 10: Saying a final goodbye.

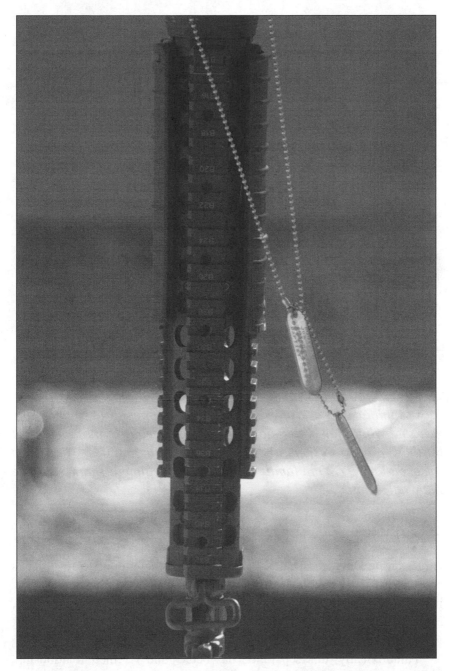

Figure 11: ID tags hang from a fallen soldier's M16 at his memorial.

- 5 -
Unpredictable, unrelenting anger

Most combat vets are angry about what happened to them in the war and what they had to do to survive it. They take that anger out on those closest to them, their wives and their families. That leads to secondary PTSD in family members, so treatment should include the whole family.

Anger drove Dave and Daneil Belcher apart, although only a few blocks apart. A married couple with a 10-year-old daughter, Katie, they now live in separate homes in Great Falls. "He needed his own separate space, somewhere he could go when he felt the anger coming on," said Daneil, who joined her husband in his apartment for our first interview.

Paradoxically, that separation has been good for their relationship. "We're much closer now than we were a few years ago," said Daneil, one stocking foot rubbing against her husband's as they try to tell me about the rage that nearly drove them apart after he got his medical discharge from the Army. Belcher served in two wars, received a head injury, and is now trying to adjust to the war-related deaths of his daughter and her fiancé a year ago.

Belcher, a former combat platoon sergeant who was awarded the Bronze Star and Combat Infantry Badge, said situations below the level of his consciousness trigger an adrenaline rush "and then I get angry, and I didn't realize I was getting there."

His wife said the Army trains soldiers to respond to unexpected situations with anger. "It's the only emotion they can use that's effective in combat," she explains. "They brainwash soldiers to react to everything with anger."

Belcher said the anger frightens him because he knows what he's capable of doing. He needs to get to a safe, quiet space because "when I get angry, I can't control it."

"Oh yes you can," Daneil contradicts. "When you get really angry, you save it for me." There's a tense moment as Belcher just stares at his wife.

"His anger is so bad that I don't even want to talk about it," said Daneil after a moment. "His anger comes out of nowhere and for no reason. And once it starts, it just gets worse, no matter what I do. So I'm scared by it. Even talking about it gives me an adrenaline rush that's twisting my gut right now."

The Belchers agree they need to talk about this problem, but that Daneil should talk to me without her husband around.

Afraid to trigger an outburst

A few days later, I visited Daneil in her home to let her angst out in private. But it was still hard for her to discuss her husband's anger because she feared she might trigger it again, even though at that moment he was driving their daughter to a skating rink with her friends. "I'm really afraid now," she said, her hands shaking gently. "He knows I'm sitting here talking about him. Three years ago, he'd have been berserk. Now they've got his meds adjusted and he hasn't blown up in two, two and one half years, but I'm still scared."

When she described her husband, she said he wasn't physically abusive — "He pushed me around a few times, but he never actually hit me." — but would explode into rage without provocation and yell at her, call her names, throw things.

"The anger is like its own entity, a separate, living and breathing creature lurking just below the surface that will wake up and roar and shoot fire, burning *me*, the safe target. Then it will go dormant, and my husband is a regular guy, a sensitive and loving husband, devoted father."

The explosions weren't just disagreements among adults, she said. "I was never able to defuse his anger. I remember wishing that I could go through one day without him calling me a 'stupid fucking bitch.' I finally realized he would only start a fight when Katie was in the room, and I think that was because he knew I wouldn't participate in the argument with our child present."

Sometimes, the only option was to leave. "I kept a bag of my stuff and Katie's stuff in the car for years," she said. "We spent the night in a motel about five times. And the really lousy part about it was that there was never an apology afterward. He would just pretend it didn't happen. It was like he didn't remember it, but I don't see how that could be."

Sometimes, however, leaving wasn't possible. Her husband would follow her around the house, yelling at her and blocking the doors, stopping her from leaving. "He never hit me, but I was always afraid he would. And he threw things at me, things like the telephone and the television channel changer. I spent a lot of time tiptoeing around, and that was wrong. It was also wrong to force Katie to be quiet. It's wrong not to let a child have a happy, normal childhood."

Reliving a nightmare

Many nights, Daneil would go to bed and lie awake, her mind racing, until her husband dropped off to sleep. Then she'd slip out to the kitchen and commit that agony to paper. Here are a few excerpts:

Dec. 6, 2004 — Ripped hair dryer out of the wall, threatened to throw it. Katie was in shower watching and crying. Called me a stupid fucking bitch in front of her.

Dec. 8, 2004 — The first week of December, the explosions came. He's intense, violent, can't stop himself once he starts yelling. He has no qualms about saying hurtful and hateful things in front of Katie. He throws things at me, lunges toward me and I'm afraid he will hurt me (Katie is frightened too as she sees this). ... I'm writing this down because I'm afraid now. Before, I didn't think he would really hurt me, but he's so strong and out of control when he's raging. I don't believe he could stop himself anymore. I don't think he'd harm Katie physically, but his behavior has to be hurting her psychologically and emotionally.

Aug. 6, 2005 — I'm losing sleep and getting headaches from the strain of living like this. Even on his good days, I'm on edge waiting for the next explosion. It always seems to come out of nowhere when I've started to believe we might be normal.... I couldn't leave when Katie was a baby because I needed to be with her. Especially when I realized I wouldn't bring any more children into "this." When she was older, I couldn't leave because I couldn't make enough money to take care of her. I'm afraid Dave would pay a lawyer to make sure Katie is taken away from me, and that terrifies me more than living like this.

Aug. 7, 2005 — Even with some sort of split custody, what would happen if he doesn't have me to yell at anymore? I don't think he'd be mean to her directly, but he'd yell about me to her and that's just as hurtful/harmful. At least if we're together, I can run interference and deflect his criticism or disapproval (when it's unreasonable) toward me instead. How sick of a relationship is that? ... If she's growing up thinking a husband can treat his wife like this, what kind of a man will she marry? Will she think it's normal to tiptoe around the house, trying not to make noise, not saying what you think or how you feel because you're afraid of setting him off? I want her to be able to express herself and assert herself with confidence, but the example I'm setting is totally the opposite. And I'm always making excuses for him to her — "It's not Daddy's fault, it's his medication." "He doesn't really hate me, he has a lot of anger from the war and this is how it comes out." "Daddy doesn't really want to leave, he's just upset about … whatever." The child [7 years old] should not have to deal with this heavy crap at such a young age.

Aug. 8, 2005 — I know there's nothing I can do to prevent this. Even if I'm perfect, he'll blow about something (even the "perfection") and I know it's not my fault, but I'm still trying to prevent it. It's so hard to have zero control over this. I keep telling myself, "He may be ruining my life, but I don't have to let him spoil my day." And I put on a happy face for Katie's sake. But I'm dying inside. I don't know who I am anymore. I keep my feelings closely guarded. I can't trust him to talk about them because he'll use them for ammo next time he attacks me. I'm afraid to have fun when we're apart, can't really relax because if I let my guard down, he hurts me worse. Katie pays the price. She should be able to laugh (and cry) and tease and play and have fun without fear of her parents. I'm always shushing her and warning her to be quiet or giving her "watch out" looks to warn her Daddy might get mad if she does her normal childhood things.

Oct. 1, 2005 — I lie in bed trying not to breathe too loudly. Sometimes I wish I wasn't breathing at all. Katie is old enough to get along without me, and I don't really have any other reason to *be*. What a relief it would be just to be done with everything....

Remembering the first (American) war in Iraq

Dave Belcher was an infantry staff sergeant during Operations Desert Shield and Desert Storm, serving on active duty from 1983 to 1995. When the Desert Storm ground war began in February 1991, Belcher's platoon with the 1st Armored Division was in the first wave to cross into Iraq and make contact with the enemy.

"It was total destruction, loss of life, and bloody," he said. "Once you go through war, it's always black and burned. One of my tracks got hit by friendly fire, and we lost one of my drivers."

The 1st Brigade of the 1st Armored Division and the 3rd Brigade of the 3rd Infantry Division were awarded the Valorous Unit Award for this engagement, which it described in military language: "On Feb. 26, the brigade was ordered to attack east to gain contact with and destroy the RGFC [Iraqi Republican Guard Forces Command] in zone. The 3rd Brigade began an aggressive and continuous movement to contact which covered 74 kilometers in 12½ hours, while fighting multiple engagements throughout the day and night, with elements of the 52nd, 17th, Adnan, and Tawakalna Divisions. During one engagement with the Tawakalna Division, the Brigade destroyed 27 Soviet T-72s [tanks] which had established a hasty defense to cover the Iraqi forces withdrawing from the Kuwaiti Theater of Operation. On Feb. 27, the 3rd Brigade was ordered to transition to pursuit operations to establish contact with and destroy the RGFC forces in zone. As the Brigade attacked and fought through the Adnan Division, securing a RGFC major logistics base, it captured 465 EPWs [enemy prisoners of war] and made contact with the Medinah Armored Division, which was augmented by elements of four other Iraqi divisions. A fierce battle ensued, culminating in the destruction of 82 tanks, 31 armored personnel carriers, 11 artillery pieces, 48 trucks, three AAA guns, and captured 72 EPWs with the loss of only two Bradley cavalry vehicles, 30 WIAs [wounded in action], and one KIA [killed in action]."

But it wasn't only long-range fighting from tanks. It was also hand-to-hand combat.

"I was also clearing trenches," said Belcher. "My job was to take my platoon and go in and kill as many of the enemy as we could." It was a dangerous job, and Belcher remembers feeling scared during the combat. "There's fear," he said, "but the adrenaline is even higher and overriding the fear." And the danger isn't always just the enemy. "Being in the trenches was very close combat. One of my guys threatened to kill me. He cocked a round, but I got his ammunition away from him and got him into counseling."

After the ground war, Belcher's battalion was assigned to provide a checkpoint to disarm people leaving Iraq and determine who would be allowed to go to Saudi Arabia as refugees. "We were checking for weapons," he said.

"And they were checking body bags to make sure they had the right stuff in them," added Daneil. Dave Belcher said, "People were trying to get out of Iraq, trying to get out of their own country because Saddam Hussein was trying to kill them or gas them. I saw a lot of dead children or burned children, but there wasn't much I could do for them."

His veterans outreach counselor, Tony Rizzo, reported on that trauma in 2003: "Mr. Belcher indicates that he observed hundreds of men, women, and children that were brutalized by the Iraqi Republican Guard or other Iraqi agencies. Many of the refugees were severely injured, including children that needed immediate medical care. Unfortunately, Mr. Belcher's unit had only a few medics to provide basic care for the refugees. The refugees would have to travel to a medical facility much farther by foot or, if lucky, by vehicle. Mr. Belcher would inspect coffins to ensure there were no guns or ammo in them. He became ill on many occasions due to the smell and sight of decomposing bodies that had been burned or torn apart by exploding ordinance. Mr. Belcher indicates that the events he witnessed while in Desert Storm have profoundly impacted his life as he has daily recollections of his combat experiences, as well as those of refugees. He especially remembers while on a convoy seeing an Iraqi woman and her two young children pleading for help because they were severely injured. Mr. Belcher wanted to stop and provide aid, but the convoy was under orders not to stop for any reason. Mr. Belcher can still see this woman's face in his mind."

Trying to mask PTSD with booze

One of his last assignments was to come to Montana to train National Guard troops in Helena, and it was there that Belcher met his wife. He left the service, married Daneil, and moved to Great Falls. He seemed normal to himself, but not to others. "I didn't know I had PTSD until I got married and had outbursts of anger at my family," he said.

Alcohol was a convenient crutch, and Belcher abused it after his discharge. "I drank a lot," he said.

Daneil added, "All day long, starting with two beers at breakfast."

"That's about right," he agreed.

But they worried that booze might be worsening his anger problem. "I was getting in a lot of bar fights," he said, so seven years ago, he stopped drinking cold turkey. "Now I don't even like the stuff."

But the outbursts of fury continued, so Belcher began seeing VA counselor, Tony Rizzo, who noted that:

"Mr. Belcher's sleep is sporadic, and he has nightmares on a regular basis of the carnage of Iraqi bodies he witnessed while in combat. He has had periods when he feels as though he was actually back in Iraq. All his senses are acute; he smells the death, hears the crying and screaming and the sounds of combat. He feels he is there and loses touch with reality until someone or something brings him back. He continues to be triggered by the sounds of children crying or screaming, even if they are only playing. Loud unexpected noises or the sight of smoke remind him of burning enemy vehicles. The sight or smell of blood or burned flesh, even barbequing, can cause him distress. He is very uncomfortable in crowds or enclosed places. He continues to feel trapped in the Bradley fighting vehicle and is terrified as though it had been hit and exploded. When he is triggered, his heart rate increases and he has panic attacks and adrenaline rushes. He becomes confused and isolates himself from others as he uses his home as a bunker or safe place."

Part of this may be due to his traumatic brain injury (TBI), which occurred when a group of robbers attacked him on base at Fort Riley,

Kansas, and knocked him unconscious with a steel bar before robbing him.

But much of it may also have been due to the trial-and-error method of adjusting his medications to get them to mask the symptoms without too many side effects.

"Sometimes he'll call me five or six times a day to ask me what day it is," said Daneil. Dave agrees, "I forget everything. It's really a terrible thing." Said Daneil, "He went to the store and bought the same things three times. The fourth time he went back, the clerk said, 'You've been here three times already for grapes and milk.'"

Even with the meds, he's still subject to flashbacks and nightmares. "I get nightmares about when we were hit by friendly fire and our guns all malfunctioned," he said. "But my worst nightmare is about killing someone. I see their faces of horror, and that's what haunts me. I know you have to kill people in war, but when you actually do it, it's something else. I'm learning the Bible now, and it said, 'Thou shalt not kill.'"

"Thou shalt not murder," I correct. "Oh, is that how they get around that one?" asks Daneil, who works as a church secretary in a Lutheran church next door to her house.

Vivid dreams of dead children also startle him awake. "The dream starts with a truckload of people, and I keep seeing burned bodies, dead bodies, burned children that I can't help. When I did the humanitarian aid, I had to deal with a lot of death, and that's what I dream about. There were a lot of kids I couldn't help, and that really hurt."

Daneil remembers her husband being very overprotective of his family. "When he first got back, he wouldn't let me leave Katie alone in the backyard," she said. "I couldn't even go into the house to go to the bathroom."

Counselor Rizzo picked up on that, too: "He is constantly on guard and has actually strung string around his yard at night to inspect the next morning to see if anyone was in his yard. He is very overprotective of his wife and daughter and does not allow his daughter to play outside unless he can see her. He gets up at night to check doors and windows or if he hears a noise outside. He is easily startled by people approaching from behind or by unexpected noises. This is one reason for his isolation in his home as it reduces exposure to contact with others and minimizes being startled."

A failed suicide attempt

Around Christmas 2003, Belcher tanked. He had known it would be dangerous to keep weapons around his own home, so he borrowed a gun and tried to shoot himself. "I couldn't take it anymore," he said. "I tried to commit suicide with my friend's gun, but I put the wrong ammunition in it, and it wouldn't fire. Otherwise I wouldn't be here today."

The next morning, his friend loaded Belcher into his pickup and drove him to the VA's regional mental health hospital in Fort Sheridan, Wyoming. It was only partially successful. "It helped me to realize that I had problems," he said. "They showed me what the problems were."

"But they didn't fix everything," added Daneil. "It wasn't the magic bullet that I had hoped it would be."

In the beginning, however, there was hope, according to Daneil's journal.

"When Dave came home from the hospital in Sheridan, he was much better," she wrote. "He was pleasant to be around. He didn't let little things irritate him. Throughout the summer, he wanted to go out and do things. He went shopping with us and took Katie to the movies. He started talking about going back to church and getting involved with Kogudus again [a Lutheran Church retreat that provides Bible studies]. I began to look forward to coming home from work instead of dreading it as I used to. My trust gradually began to build up again. Six months was way beyond any other time he'd been 'normal.'"

Through that fall, there were a few times when Belcher got angry, but there was none of the explosive rage that his family had been used to. But in October, his medications were changed, and he responded badly. "He was having double vision and seeing people that weren't there," said Daneil. Then he began getting quieter and progressively more tense.

That became the pattern for the next several years. The explosive rages would send him back to the VA doctors seeking help. They'd adjust his meds, and that would alleviate the problem. With her husband calmer, Daneil would gradually, very gradually, allow herself to hope that they might have a stable household again. Then Belcher's meds would be adjusted again — the last time was to switch out an antidepressant that might cause subsequent joint problems — and the fury would return. Finally, Daneil could take it no longer.

"This time when he threatened to leave, I agreed with him and told him he should, as I just cannot live like this anymore," she wrote in her diary. "Even when he's not sullen and angry, I'm constantly on edge, watching for signs and trying to prevent a blowup. But I've finally realized I can do nothing to prevent it or to diffuse it once it begins. If I agree with everything he says, it still escalates. If I do everything right, he gets mad at me for being perfect. He tells me I make him mad on purpose when I'm doing everything I can to not trigger it."

Separate housing helps

So Belcher moved into a furnished apartment a few blocks away from his home. He sleeps there most nights, and he goes there when he's beginning to feel tense. To avoid triggers, Belcher avoids most social situations and crowds. He tries to go to church with his wife, but feels out of place due to the guilt associated with his combat experiences. And he tries to avoid going near the oil refinery in Great Falls because "It smells just like war. I get this adrenaline rush, and then I get angry without realizing it."

Now he faces a whole new problem, the war-related deaths of his daughter from a previous marriage and her fiancé. "My daughter hung herself last year because her fiancé got killed by a roadside bomb in Iraq," he said. "She was just 19."

Laura Elizabeth Belcher died October 16, 2006, and her dad is still stunned by it. His meds numb some of the pain, but never quite enough. "If I hadn't been on meds, I don't know what would have happened," he said. "When I got that phone call, I just couldn't understand it. And when we went to the funeral, my dad and brothers went with me to help me because I just couldn't function. My other daughter is taking it real hard, too, because she's the one who found her body. It's hard for her to keep a job now, so I send her a little money."

To help him get through the ordeal, Belcher has been taking a Bible study class, although his short-term memory loss makes it difficult for him to remember what he has just read. Frequently, he'll read a passage over and over again. But he finds a peace in it. "After I tried to kill myself and failed, I decided to turn my life over to God," he said.

"Our life is so much better now, but it still feels like a delicate balance to me," said Daneil. "His involvement in his VA group [Vets4Vets] and his Bible study have done wonders. He still is uncomfortable in small crowds, but he doesn't completely avoid them anymore or let them work him up."

Secondary PTSD among families

While Belcher will probably require counseling and medication for the rest of his life, his family shares the strain. "I think I have secondary PTSD from what I've been through with Dave," said Daneil. "Families of the vets need help, too, a lot more than what we've been getting. There ought to be a support group just for spouses, but I don't know that it would do any good. All the vets who are in denial are so paranoid they'd never let their wives go to a group like that. I know that up until a few years ago, I'd never have dared go, no matter how much I needed it. The insanity of this whole thing now is that he's so much better — he hasn't exploded at me in several years — but I can't get over it."

I told Daneil that she needed counseling to help her get over the anxiety and anger that are tormenting her, and I gave her the name of a counselor, a bright and understanding woman with whom I've worked over the years. At first she said she was afraid, that she'd think about it. But a couple of months later, Belcher sought me out at our Bible study class. "Daneil's going to a counselor, and it seems to be helping," he said. "I'm really glad she's doing it."

Several months later, however, I asked Daneil about the counseling. "I can't bring myself to go," she said. "I know I need it, and my pastor recommended counseling — in fact she recommended the same counselor — but I just keep thinking that if I can make it through this day, it'll be OK."

That's just an excuse, and Daneil knows it. She's afraid to face her problems. She's carrying a huge load of anger and fear, and she needs professional help to stave off major illness. What's worse, I know there are many, many women suffering in silence who need that help and more.

Seeking help in New York City

Anger was also the problem that former Spec. Rob Timmons of New York City brought back from his 11-month deployment with the 101st Airborne. I talked with Timmons when I visited the Iraq and Afghanistan Veterans of America in lower Manhattan at the end of a visit to New York City in 2007 to judge the Pulitzer Prizes.

"I was infantry, so I was kicking down doors, escorting fuel trucks, patrolling villages and towns," he said. "We were cops, social workers, medics, doing a variety of roles."

Despite his training, though, the first sight of death stunned him.

"I came across the body of a girl, perhaps 10 to 12 years old, in a building we had been searching," said Timmons. "I had prepared myself for the sight of a dead Iraqi man in uniform, but this was a young girl in a bright dress and her body was decomposing. It was the first dead body I'd ever seen, and the sight stayed with me for a long time."

But war came closer when members of Timmons's unit, including his closest drinking buddy, were killed in a firefight. "By the time I got there, medics were picking up body parts, including someone's arm. I found out later that a good buddy of mine had been killed there."

The next day, Timmons was providing guard duty for a convoy, which meant that he and his Humvee blocked off a cross street until the convoy had passed through. But there was one truck that kept inching up on him, refusing to stop. "I kept yelling at him to stop, but he wouldn't," said Timmons. "Finally, I pointed my weapon at him. He just pointed to his forehead, as if to say, 'Shoot me here.' I was thinking about my dead friend, and I got enraged. I went up to the window of his truck, felt for my bayonet because I was thinking about cutting his throat, but it was back in my Humvee so I grabbed the butt of my rifle and started beating on him. It was a primal rage. I just lost it there, and I can't quit thinking about it."

Coming home Rob was a difficult adjustment. "At first, I couldn't sleep at all. Then after the excitement of being home wore off, the insomnia remained. I was also hyperactive. I would look at every situation, watch all the trucks, and check out every exit in a building. I couldn't get within 200 feet of a crowd, which is a huge problem in New York City. One time, I heard the sound of a beer distributor dropping his load and I almost tackled my girlfriend to get her to the ground where it was safe. I was troubled by a lot of recurring thoughts."

The rage Timmons experienced in Iraq came back recently when he was helping a friend move out of an apartment and the landlord was ugly and threatening. Timmons walked away from an altercation, but realized his anger was a problem. He called the VA for help and was told an appointment for an evaluation would take 45 days.

"They're overstretched, underfunded, and understaffed," said Timmons, who is struggling to understand how war has changed him. "I was a laidback guy, but ever since my deployment, high-stress situations make me feel like I have to protect people. And, unfortunately, I either deal with it through verbal muscle or through a wish to use violence. The infantry culture is to identify a threat and eliminate it. But it's different back home, and a lot of men and women have a lot of trouble making the transition.

"If I'm not busy, if I have a moment to breathe, I dwell on my combat experiences. So I try to spend my time with friends, family, and work. When I'm not busy, I can't relax," he concluded.

Trying to defuse the anger

Anger is a huge issue for most combat vets. Some therapists say anger is the mirror image of fear. If you can show a vet there's no longer a reason for that constant state of fear, you can also begin to defuse the anger. But the anger can also come from the futility of war, from the senseless loss of life all around you, and that's a more difficult issue to deal with because there's no rational solution other than the Serenity Prayer ("God, grant me the serenity to accept the things I cannot change, courage to change the things I can, and wisdom to know the difference.").

But a vet needs to understand that blowing up at his family and friends is a misplaced emotion. His anger should be directed at the things that affected him in wartime, and his efforts should be directed at changing his thought patterns and identifying his current triggers so that he can control their reactions. Doing both will allow his pool of rage to be reduced. And there are a number of techniques that can be useful. One is called *safe-place imagery*, which encourages a vet to focus on a key image that gives him or her a sense of security when stress begins to build. Like kids, some may need a timeout from an emotion that threatens to overwhelm them. A place to go to be alone and wind down can be invaluable, as the Belchers are finding.

A Marine colonel's tragedy

War profoundly changed the personality and the life of former reserve Marine Lt. Col. Mike Zacchea, who now works as a commodities analyst for a major Wall Street brokerage firm in Westchester, New York, and lives just across the state line in Brookfield, Connecticut.

Marcy Zacchea told me she remembers meeting her husband-to-be on a train six years ago. "He just started talking with me, a total stranger. He was extremely social, a very likeable guy who could talk with anyone. He's very intelligent. He has a great heart, generous. And he was very athletic, in great shape."

They began dating before he left for Iraq. "He was great, funny," she said. "We never fought, ever."

Iraq changed that.

"When he came back, he was withdrawn, which was a big change," Marcy said. "He also had this sadness in his eyes. It seemed to me like he was lost. I've seen that look in other guys, and once you see it, you immediately recognize it. When Mike had been home less than six months, someone stopped him on the street and said he hadn't seen that thousand-year stare in years. He asked if Mike needed help, but Mike said something rude to him.

"I was living in an apartment then, and Mike would come to see me. Once we started to fight. He cursed me and smashed a wall. I knew I had to leave, so I went out and sat in my car for an hour — it was cold — before I finally went back in."

As a condition of getting married, Marcy insisted they both go to counseling. It was an ultimatum that she regrets having to make, but one that was absolutely necessary, she said.

"He gets this look in his eye, and that's what scares me the most," said Marcy. "It's a weird look, like there's a monster in there. I never know what's going to set it off, so I've learned to tippytoe and be real careful when I bring things up. After we were married (about two years ago), he was still very involved with keeping in touch with the people back in Iraq, and he found out one of his Iraqi interpreters had been killed. We got into a terrible fight, and he started throwing things. I tried to lock myself in the bathroom, but I couldn't because he was right behind me. I was afraid he was going to hit me, so I brought my hand up in self-defense, but he didn't hit me. Finally he left, and I locked the door. There was a lot of noise out there, so I stayed in the bathroom for about an hour. When it quieted down, I opened the door and found it blocked by a bunch of furniture and chairs and boxes and things. I finally pushed the stuff out of the way and got out. There was stuff everywhere that he'd thrown, and I refused to pick it up."

After a few days, Zacchea finally apologized and began cleaning up the mess, according to Marcy.

"I was very, very aggressive and got into a lot of physical altercations with people, some of whom deserved it and some didn't," said Zacchea. "I was very, very lucky not to get arrested. I deserved it on several occasions."

One of those occasions convinced Zacchea that he needed help, he told me. "I destroyed the house on several occasions, and when I was buying flowers for my wife, I got into an altercation with the clerk. She was trying to close up and didn't want to make change for me, and I was very aggressive. She finally threw the change at me, and I caught it in my left hand and grabbed her throat with my right hand and started to squeeze," he said. "That frightened her, and it frightened me. I ran out of the store."

That's abnormal behavior for a medically disabled reserve Marine Corps lieutenant colonel who has won two Bronze Stars for valor in combat. "To me, PTSD means a combat response to a civilian provocation," Zacchea said. "And it's totally inappropriate behavior."

Zacchea has lived through the worst of combat

To understand that behavior, you have to understand that Zacchea has been through some of the worst combat experiences that a human being can be asked to endure. And that has scarred him, probably permanently.

Zacchea was in combat in both Somalia and Haiti, but he said they were inconsequential because he never felt the ongoing sense of desperation that he felt in Iraq. As senior battalion advisor to the 5th Battalion, 3rd Brigade of the Iraqi 5th Division, he was trying to train an Iraqi battalion that started out with roughly 900 soldiers and officers, many of whom had never been in the military before. No place was safe, not even their base, al-Taji, which is just north of Baghdad.

"We had a bombing in our dining facility on August 26 [2004], and five were killed and 22 wounded," Zacchea says. "The American advisors used to have a meeting at the end of the day, but my friend [Iraqi major] Saeed had come to pick me up and we were going to have dinner together. We were just walking out and heard the explosion and saw the smoke column 400 or 500 meters away. We were among the first on the scene. The dining hall was blown to hell, and there were a bunch of dead and wounded lying around. The Iraqis need to gather every bit of flesh so they can bury it, and I have this very vivid memory of the Iraqis shoulder to shoulder, crawling through the muck and blood to gather these bits of flesh on shards of glass. After a couple of hours, Saeed decided not to eat, but as he was getting in his truck, he pointed out that I had a bit of flesh on my boot. That made me vomit. They were making curried chicken, and to this day I cannot smell any kind of curry without beginning to gag."

The success of the dining hall bomb unnerved the Iraqi soldiers, said Zacchea, and more than 100 of them quickly deserted. Adding to their unrest was a constant threat of being captured by the insurgents and beheaded.

"We were at a base camp about 10 miles north of Baghdad," Zacchea continued. "The insurgents had set up an illegal checkpoint there and had interdicted and beheaded a number of Iraqi contractors. We received a mission to recover the bridge and prevent them from doing that again. We secured the area and established a presence there randomly so they would never know when we would be there. The insurgents try to punish any tactical success, so they began infiltrating our base with snipers. Then they made a fairly large assault on the base September. 13 [2004]. I went out, immediately came under machine gun fire, and crashed my vehicle in a ditch. Everyone believed I'd been hit in the hail of gunfire. When I ran back to base, I was tackled and my flak jacket was torn off to see where I'd been hit. Ultimately, I called in air strikes, and we destroyed them."

Shortly after three contractors, two American and one British, were abducted and beheaded just outside their base, Zacchea also received a death threat in Arabic: "The dog Zacchea will die like the other infidels." His friend Saeed, a member of the al-Jubouri tribe, countered the threat by adopting Zacchea into his tribe and telling other members of the battalion that anyone who harmed a hair on Zacchea's head would be killed.

The sniper infiltrations continued about every other night, however, and Zacchea remembers them as simply terrifying. "Around the base, there were a lot of destroyed buildings and rubble and abandoned warehouses. They would lure us into those buildings to negate our night vision goggles that work on ambient light. It's black in there, and you can't see a thing. There are bullets going by you, both in front and in back. The Iraqis are notoriously poor shots, so I was constantly expecting to be shot from the front, from the back, or from any other direction. It's completely nerve wracking because you can see the blasts and hear the high-pitched whine of bullets going past you. My senses became incredibly acute as I tried to see through the dark. I was sensitive to the slightest sound, smell, change in wind or temperature. It's like the difference between regular TV and high-definition TV — all my senses were high-definition."

The sniper infiltrations stopped after Zacchea's unit took the offensive September 29. "We did a raid on the mosque in al-Mousafura,

captured 51 insurgents and what up until then was the largest weapons
cache in Iraq. It was pretty textbook. We caught them at morning prayers
about 5:30, and they gave up without a fight. They had all the weapons
and bombs right there. That was a big coup, and the area calmed down a
lot after that."

An even bigger challenge

From there, the unit was sent to Fallujah, the insurgent stronghold, and
that order precipitated more disruptions. It was an administrative
nightmare because the Iraqi soldiers threw away their Army ID cards as
fast as the advisors could make them, Zacchea said. "When I announced
where we were going, there were riots, both for and against. A couple of
days later, three quarters of the Iraqi battalion had deserted, and I was
devastated. Many had abandoned their guard posts to leave, so that made
us even more vulnerable. The specter of failure loomed large for our
advisor team and the battalion. Later, they began to come back, saying
they had been taking their stuff home and saying goodbye to their
families!"

It was a 40-mile drive to Fallujah, and "We were under fire most of
the way," Zacchea said. "We had one killed, 16 wounded, and we lost
four vehicles running the gauntlet. It reminded me of the road to Hell."

The Marines and Iraqi soldiers were expected to retake Fallujah, but
there was an immediate setback. "Right before the assault, one of my
company commanders deserted with the battle plans, and I had to go to
the commanding general and brief him. That was very, very
disconcerting and embarrassing."

But the attack went on as planned. "The city was under mortar fire
all night and getting pounded. It was a stormy night, and we had AC-130
gunships coming in and pounding the city. Artillery was pounding the
city. It was pretty dramatic." In the craziness, Zacchea remembers an
amphibious assault vehicle struck by incoming fire with Marines
tumbling out on fire, all shredded up and screaming. In the midst of it
was a Marine sergeant major demanding that his men tough it out.

"The city was breached at dawn [November 8, 2004]," Zacchea said.
"We were going door to door, getting into brutal fights, house to house

and room to room, particularly in the stairways of buildings that are basically death funnels. I did enough of that to know that I never want to do it again. Some of our guys who did that hundreds of times have my undying admiration because you have no idea how difficult that was."

On the fourth day of pitched fighting, Zacchea was wounded. "We were assaulting a house and started taking machine gun fire from another house down the street. Three other Marines and I advanced on the machine gun nest and bounded over a wall. Two of us were firing our rifles as the third threw a hand grenade in the window. He turned around, and his eyes got wide as he saw an RPG [rocket-propelled grenade] team on a rooftop behind us. I was closest and chose to engage them while the other Marines ran for cover. I was firing on them when they shot the RPG right at me. I could see it and hear it coming. It exploded just behind me, and I went up in the air."

When two of the Marines got him out of there, Zacchea saw that he had taken shrapnel in the shoulder so extensive that his shoulder blade was broken. "I bled for a week, couldn't raise my arm over my head, but it was important for me to show up for duty again. They recommended medevaccing me to a combat surgical hospital, but I declined so they gave me some painkillers and I got about 12 hours of sleep. Then the next morning, I was back in the fight. When I came back again, that really motivated the Iraqis."

When it was all over, Zacchea found he had no sympathy for their vanquished foe. "We had a lot of insurgents who were dying and came to us for help," he said. "There was a lot of despair in them for having to come to us for help. Allah wouldn't save them. They'd been lied to and deceived. And I have to be honest — I really enjoyed their despair and their suffering, both physical and emotional. I thought it was just and right that they should suffer. We found multiple dead bodies in their homes, people who had been tortured and beheaded in their homes. Ninety percent of the vehicles in that city had been rigged to explode. It was a brutal fight, and the insurgents were brutal to us and brutal to each other."

Zacchea was awarded a Bronze Star for that episode, which also won him the respect and trust of his Iraqi battalion. But that trust turned out to be a bittersweet blessing.

"Right before Christmas 2004, we let the battalion out on leave," he said. "They came back at the end of January, and things were chaotic. Several of our soldiers had been abducted and beheaded. Others had been abducted and tortured and sent back to us. We had to have our military intelligence people debrief them, and the soldiers would not speak with them without me being present. It was harrowing being there with them as they talked about being beaten and burned and electrocuted and whipped and drilled and all the other things those people do to each other."

Sitting through those accounts of brutal torture was like being raped, said Zacchea.

One ordeal remained. Six weeks or so before he was scheduled to return home, an Iraqi soldier came to him privately with details of an assassination attempt. "We did a sting operation and caught them as they were putting the plot into motion," he said. "There was a court-martial and the soldiers involved were sentenced to 30 days in our own brig, then dismissed from the army. The insurgent was also court-martialed and sentenced to 45 days in our brig on bread and water. Shortly before I left, he disappeared and I don't know what happened to him. I don't know if he was executed or let out — anything could have happened to him. But I suspect he was executed because our battalion commander told me as I was leaving, 'Don't look too closely into this.'"

Acing the tests for PTSD

After the assassination attempt, Zacchea said he sought help from the combat stress clinic. "They asked me a whole bunch of questions, and I popped a positive on every one of them. They asked me how many firefights I'd been in, and I estimated 85 to 100 firefights. The psych said I should have seen him long before, but I never had the time to do it."

Coming home only revealed the damage that his adrenaline had been hiding from himself and from others. "I couldn't eat, couldn't sleep, and was having nightmares. My wife insisted on my seeing a counselor. She said I kept saying, 'I can't stay here! I've got to get out of here!' I basically have no memory of the first five months I was home."

Zacchea said he knew substance abuse would be deadly, so he avoided drinking. But the Fourth of July put him back in country. "The first July 4, I went into my basement and barricaded myself, set up a defensive position in my basement." He was also a defensive driver, to the horror of others on the road. "When I was driving, I'd see things on the side of the road or hear noises and react like I was in combat. I'd swerve like I was avoiding an IED. I'm usually driving 80 or 90 miles an hour. The only defense is speed in Iraq. If you slow down, you're dead."

Zacchea is still geared for combat in Connecticut and in New York. "My reflexes are very fast, and I notice everything. I'm constantly scanning rooftops and windows for activity. I've gotten into a number of confrontations because my fight-or-flight mechanism is so extreme that it happens without my realizing it."

And he's still grappling with the root cause of his anger and how he can shut it off or turn it down. "I think one of the causes is the personal betrayal, the people who deserted in the face of the enemy, or the people who absconded with the battalion payroll in Fallujah, which would have cost us our mission if the Iraqis went home because we couldn't pay them. Also, I killed a lot of people, and there's a lot of anger and grief over that. And there's a lot of anger and outrage about our Iraqi soldiers being abducted and tortured. We discovered a number of grotesque and profoundly disturbing videos. It's hard to describe how awful that was. They filmed Iraqis being beheaded, being profoundly tortured before being beheaded. It was outrageous. It violated every principle of human dignity I was ever taught. Those things profoundly affected me."

Loss of memory and loss of balance

Marcy Zacchea is concerned about her husband's memory loss. "We went to see a friend about four months after he got back. A year later, we went back and he had absolutely no recollection of ever having been there. I had to convince him that he'd been there by bringing other people over and asking them whether they remembered meeting Mike a year before, and they all did."

He's had C-T scans to determine whether he suffered traumatic brain injury. Although they've found nothing, Zacchea knows something is wrong. "I've been falling down a lot, six times in the past month, and that's something that's never happened to me before," he said. "What I'm doing, I'm doing in spite of the VA, not with them."

Zacchea is gradually pulling himself together with the help of a local Vet Center. "No one thing works for me, but it all works together. I don't think there's a comprehensive solution. I've had to do it all myself — individual counseling, group counseling, medication, and working with other vets."

Now Zacchea reads everything he can find about Iraq, watches all the movies, and talks with other vets about it. "I'm really obsessed with trying to understand Iraq and my role in it," he said.

Making life a little more difficult is the fact that Zacchea heard that Jack, the loyal Iraqi who alerted him to that assassination attempt, was in danger of losing his own life. Jack was brought to America, and he is living with the Zaccheas. Asked how his wife was tolerating that, there was a brief silence. Finally, he sighed, "not well."

But Marcy said the problem was not with Jack, but with the way her husband went about the whole situation. "He told me that Jack was coming to live with us, and if I didn't like it, I could leave. After Jack came, I told Mike that if this ever happens again, I *will* leave. And he apologized for the way he handled that situation."

Zacchea said having Jack in the house set him back a little, and his wife agrees. "In October when Jack came, I noticed the rage coming back," said Marcy. "He kicked the door in once, and he took a knife to a pillow."

Shortly after that, the doctors changed Zacchea's medications, and the new meds seem to be stabilizing him a little better, she said. But, she notes, they'd be lost if Zacchea didn't have a decent job and private insurance. "We're paying to go to private doctors because you can't wait for the VA," said Marcy. "Nothing happens as the months go by, and you lose your eligibility. And you can't wait when you're in crisis. The VA needs to be doing much more for these men and women who go to war and come back completely different, physically and emotionally. I don't know how a vet can do it without good insurance, but if you can't hold a job, you don't have insurance. We're lucky Mike can still hold a job."

Marcy said her husband has put on a lot of weight; he no longer exercises because it hurts too much. And she's not sure whether the passage of time or talking about the trauma will prove to be most therapeutic in the long run.

"I realize he's handling a lot of things now, and because he's my husband, I'm handling them, too," Marcy said. "I wonder sometimes whether because I accept these things, he'll begin to think they're acceptable. But he always feels remorse and apologizes, so I have to accept it.

"No one could have expected what this war would do to Mike," Marcy said. "I had no idea what he'd come home like, and neither did he. Never in a million years would I have expected what happened to him over there."

Zacchea thinks that's a statement the federal government should take to heart. "The VA tells us that we're supposed to self-identify for PTSD, but that's wrong," he explained. "Everybody should be treated for PTSD. I think 100 percent of the people who have been under fire or fired on others potentially have PTSD. Instead of assuming that everyone's OK unless they can prove otherwise, I think it ought to be the other way around."

Recently, Zacchea was tested again for traumatic brain injury, and the results were positive. That gives him a double disability, and both are likely to be permanent. He tells me he has no regrets about his decision to serve, but I find myself haunted by the image of a retired Marine Corps colonel running from a flower shop where he's just tried to strangle a young clerk. What's wrong with this picture?

As a nation, we need to be looking at what we are doing to the soldiers we're sending into combat all around the globe. Some don't survive, but most of the ones who do come home will be changed forever. I don't think we've fully grasped that point yet. And I have to agree with Zacchea that the VA should assume every soldier who goes to war will come back traumatized and automatically provide help until the soldier feels it's no longer needed.

- 6 -
Home but alone

Not all wives can stand the strain of separation, the constant fear of a battlefield death, or even the return of a dramatically changed spouse. Divorce rates are much higher than the norm, so the Face of Combat may be a loner.

When the doors clanged shut on the DC-10 in Kuwait, the mood changed instantly. Soldiers from the Montana National Guard's 163rd Infantry Battalion had survived a year of fighting in Iraq, and they were finally headed home. Soldiers who hadn't been speaking to each other were now chatting or playing games together. "Some of them were a little worse for wear, but we brought 'em all home," remembers Sgt. 1st Class Calvin James, platoon sergeant for Company B, which was based in Great Falls.

It had been a tough year for this infantry battalion because there was no place and no time that a soldier could let his guard down and relax. "I lost count of the number of times snipers shot at me," James said. "I quit counting at 72 or 73. And I never could catch him or get a shot back at the son of a bitch because I was never able to see him. It got so that once that bastard fired his obligatory two rounds at me, I could relax for the rest of the day knowing there wouldn't be any more shots at my team."

With death always a heartbeat away, James had to disassociate himself from constant fear. "In a situation like that, you have to accept it for what it is and tell yourself that it doesn't matter. Once the bullet hits the wall beside you, it's too late to duck. You have to set your fear aside because if you don't, you'll be like a rabbit, afraid of his own shadow."

But refusing to acknowledge a legitimate emotion also sets up future emotional problems. "An infantry soldier cannot go through what we went through and not come home without PTSD," said James, one of many who have been diagnosed with post-traumatic stress disorder, as well as traumatic brain injury.

As the plane droned back to the states, James kept remembering the day he lost a dozen of the Iraqi soldiers he was in charge of training. They were his "Iraqi kids," as distinguished from the "American kids" in his platoon, and he was attached to both. Moreover, as their sergeant, he was responsible for both.

As he was driving outside of al-Hawijah, the first of three VBIEDs went off right behind him. Called vehicle-borne improvised explosive devices, these are basically car bombs. "VBIEDs went off at three of our checkpoints with massive casualties," said James. "I lost 12 or 13 of our Iraqi soldiers, and I don't know how many other civilians. When something that big hits, they literally bring in bags full of body parts and muck and goo. That first VBIED missed me by about 20 seconds. The radios began to go crazy as we continued driving to the Iraqi Army compound. Shortly after pulling into the compound two more blasts rocked the city from the northern and western checkpoints in what was obviously a coordinated attack. A passing patrol from B Co. and my team quickly secured the local hospital across the road from the Iraqi Army compound, and my team medic SSgt. Dean Sowers and the patrol Combat Life Savers began working on casualties as ambulances started arriving. There were also cars and trucks bringing people in with catastrophic injuries. We literally had a room full of bodies and body parts. They brought in men and women and kids, as well as parts of a number of Iraqi soldiers that I could recognize."

It was painful for James to see the carnage, particularly the soldiers he had been developing camaraderie with. "Later that night, when I had some time to think about what had just happened, it was overwhelming — but not totally overwhelming because we had lost some other people in battle who were old friends of mine. But it surely gets to guys who have a wife and kids back home and who have to deal with dead women or a kid coming in in eight or nine pieces, all wrapped up in a blanket."

James is a big guy, 250 pounds of muscle wrapped on a six-foot frame, and sitting for hours in a rigid plane seat only made his back feel worse. It had been hurting pretty badly for the entire tour of duty due to a compressed disk that he'd suffered while in training camp in Fort Bliss, Texas. "It began to bother me right after we began taking simulated sniper fire and I dove into a gutter. As near as I can figure, that's when I broke my back. A lot of it was because I'd been issued a flak jacket that was too small for me, and it put my body in an unnatural position."

Long-distance relationship

Naturally, James yearned to see his wife, Brendalee, again. They'd been married a year before his unit was deployed, but they emailed each other on almost a daily basis. In fact, shortly after he left, she wrote this poem:

> Ever so far away my mind does wonder and dream.
> Forever it has been since his hand held mine it may seem.
> Days come and go I can't decipher one from the other,
>   they are
> all the same. Is it reality or another dream?
>
> I remember him holding me tight.
> We laughed and snuggled through the night.
> The military called him and he went to fulfill
> his patriotic duty. He made a promise to his men
> to take them there and back again.

So each morning I arise and take care of his chores and
    mine,
then to work a day or 8 hours or maybe 9.
Back home I travel, feeding the horses and doing the
    chores.
I once waited for nightfall, but no more.
Night comes vividly and makes me aware of
time and I know I am alone. I go to the calendar and
mark off another day. I etch it like in stone.

I have never been more proud nor stood more tall
than to know my husband proudly serves this land.
His granddaughter grows and learns without him,
however, no different than the men and their children.
They dream and worship their hero's they are the men.

They bring us freedom, they bring us praise,
they allow us to sleep,
they allow us with the flag they raise.
So for tonight my dear, as with every other,
I send my love as does my children, your siblings, your
    father
and your mother….

We love you and we stand beside you.

Closer to home

Finally, their plane touched down in Fort Lewis, Washington "They told
us welcome home, but we weren't home yet," said James. "We had to go
through debriefings and medical checks. We knew that if we answered
yes to any of those questions, we'd be held back for a week or two, so we
answered no to everything because we wanted to see our wives and
children as soon as we could."

Two days before their arrival, James said he called Brendalee and she promised to take the day off from work and meet him at the airport. "When we took off from Fort Lewis, you could feel the relief in the air," he said. "And when we touched down in Great Falls, I was afraid our guys were going to tear the windows out of the airplane because they were so anxious to see their families who were all lined up there to greet them."

James scanned the crowd for his wife, but couldn't see her. His mom and his sister were there, and they embraced him. His sister, Robin Sainsbury, told him she'd called Brendalee about an hour before and been assured she was en route to the airport from their ranch home just outside Helena, about 100 miles southwest of Great Falls. "She had told me she'd pick me up at the airport, but she wasn't there. I was worried about her. Had she been in an accident, hit a deer?" wondered James. "But I was trying to hold all that back and keep track of my men."

With jubilant families all around him, James called the Montana Highway Patrol to see if there'd been a wreck on the Interstate. No wreck, they told him.

"I was relieved and grateful to be back home, but we had one more dog and pony show to go through, a big parade through town on our buses," said James. "Our guys were having fits about it because they just wanted to go home and be with their wives and families."

James kept looking out the window of his bus, but his wife wasn't there. "All of my thoughts were on my wife," he said. "She was a borderline diabetic and then had told me she had been diagnosed with lupus, so I called the sheriff's office and asked them to go out to the house and make sure she was OK." Later, the sheriff called back to say no one was at the house. But she wasn't at the National Guard Armory where the company was lined up in a stand-down ceremony and dismissed.

"I was feeling really lost," said James. "I had walked off the plane filled with joy at being able to see my wife, but that turned into the anguish of not having her there." So he finally asked his brother-in-law, Bob Sainsbury, for a lift home. "We thought there's got to be a reason," said Sainsbury. "Something's happened. So I was checking the side of the road for her car."

An empty house

When they got home, however, James knew immediately that something was seriously wrong. "I walked up to the house with a big lump in my throat, but it was empty. I looked inside and I saw a bunch of stuff was missing. I saw that my dog had been left in the house with a 50-pound sack of dog food, drinking out of an open toilet and crapping on the floor. The whole house smelled like dog shit."

For three days, James was in shock. No one knew where his wife was and she didn't call. He tried to clean the house, but it just made him furious. He couldn't handle seeing all the other things around the house that had been so neglected. "Then after a few days, I discovered the phone bill and the electric bill hadn't been paid in about six months. The house payment hadn't been paid in six months either, and the bank was fixing to foreclose on it."

With mounting anxiety, James made a trip to the bank where he'd been sending all his combat-duty paychecks. "I had $47,500 in that bank account and it was all gone. That really put me in a huge financial hole. I had to watch every nickel. I couldn't go downtown to have a burger with my buddies because I couldn't afford it. I had to borrow the money from my dad to divorce her. She just destroyed my life for a while."

To this day, James said he hasn't seen Brendalee or heard from his former wife. She didn't show up for the divorce proceedings, and deputies were never able to find her to serve a subpoena. "I spent a few months wondering about what had happened, but now I don't give a shit," he said.

None of the family saw it coming either, said his sister Robin. "He idolized her and was completely stunned that she wasn't there. And the rest of the family was equally stunned. It's really shaken us all up."

War pulls families apart

The war in Iraq has put a tremendous strain on military families. A study of new veterans referred to the VA for behavioral health evaluation found that two-thirds of the married or cohabiting veterans reported some kind of family adjustment problems, while 56 percent reported conflicts involving "shouting, pushing, or shoving." Reports of infidelity grew from four percent in 2003-05 to 14 percent in 2006 and 15 percent in 2007. Similarly, 11 percent of the soldiers said they were planning a divorce in 2003-05, but that number increased to 15 percent in 2006 and 20 percent in 2007. The Mental Health Advisory Team IV's final report concluded that 27 percent of deployed soldiers admitted marital problems.

Those problems are shared by the children. More than 700,000 children have had a parent deployed at some point during the conflict. Almost 19,000 children have had a parent wounded in action, and 2,200 children have lost a parent in Iraq or Afghanistan. A study by the Army's Family Advocacy Program suggests the deployments may also have led to a dramatic increase in the amount of child abuse in military families. It examined reports of neglect and abuse within 1,771 military families with nearly 3,000 children and found child neglect was almost four times greater in periods when the husband was deployed; physical child abuse was about double. The results of that study are consistent with earlier research showing that child neglect within Army families increased sharply after the terrorist attacks of September 11, 2001, reversing a decade-long downward trend.

Soldiers can also come apart

"This happens more often than you would think," said James. "A lot of guys come home and discover their families are gone and strangers are living in their house."

Since then, the responsible first sergeant has slowly come apart, trying to hold onto his job despite outbursts of anger. At a Post-Deployment Health Reassessment Task Force meeting in Helena, James said he was applying for a medical discharge with PTSD being a prime component. "I was urged to come here by my chaplain, but I was asked not to come here and air our dirty laundry by my chain of command," he said.

But applying for a disability is foreign to his nature. "It makes me feel like a whiner because I'm the guy other people come to with their problems," he said. The National Guard's response to his plight has made him even more bitter. "When I was in Iraq, I was tasked with training the Iraqi Army," he told the task force. "And I was treated better by the Iraqi Army than I have been by the Montana National Guard."

He's free to speak out because he has more than 20 years in service and can retire at any time with good pay and benefits. But younger soldiers with less time in service can be thrown off active duty for speaking out, which will cost them their GI benefits, including a college education and medical benefits, he said. "A lot of these guys won't talk with anyone because they're afraid of losing their benefits."

With the difficulty the returning soldiers are having, they can't afford to lose those benefits. "Some of our guys have changed jobs, gotten divorces, or gotten into trouble for running people off the road," said James. "I'd guess 75 to 80 percent of our guys are having trouble fitting in or having family troubles. A lot of guys are over there, serving multiple tours because they don't fit in at home anymore. One of our guys is on his third tour. He served with us in Iraq, came home, and found out that he didn't fit in anymore so he volunteered to go back. When he came home a second time, he found out that his wife had moved out to California with her new boyfriend, so he went back for his third tour.

"If my dad's health weren't so bad, I'd probably be over there again myself," he added. "Sometimes it's easier to have a guy honestly trying to kill you than to have to put up with all this bureaucratic bullshit."

Huge burden on the family

It should be no surprise that relationships fail during and after deployments. When a soldier is home, he plays an active role with his wife and family. He's likely to be in the stands when his kids play baseball, cleaning up the kitchen after dinner, mowing the grass, or paying the bills. But when he heads off to war, those responsibilities fall to his wife and kids. Then when he comes home, he may be an entirely different person, someone that they don't know. But even if he were to be completely unchanged, the whole dynamic of his family relationship has changed in his absence and he needs to find a way to fit in again.

Think of a family as a mobile, cardboard cutouts hanging on threads and moving together in intricate patterns as a gentle breeze blows. When one of those figures is removed, the entire dynamic changes. And at its simplest, that's what happens when the soldier disappears ... and when he returns.

Across the country, National Guard commanders are beginning to understand that soldiers returning from combat need to have some time where they can be together with each other, but also with their families. Some states have begun to schedule the first weekend drill in a motel where families can talk or socialize. A summer weekend picnic would serve the same purpose. There needs to be a time to relax, to talk, and to begin to understand what's been happening to dad while he's been gone ... and what has happened to his family during that time, too.

Montana is beginning to adopt that model, as we will see in chapter 16, and it's a wise choice. A soldier is much stronger if he has a supportive family behind him.

- 7 -
Booze and nightmares

Faces reflected in bottles of booze are also Faces of Combat. From World War II to Iraq we find faces hoping that alcohol or other self-medication will help, and discovering that it won't.

In December of 1969, when Robert King came home from the war in Vietnam, he crawled into a whiskey bottle for relief.

"My nightmares came all night long, and when I woke up in the morning, I'd be worn out," he said. "I'd dream about those Viet Cong in their black pajamas, coming to get me. They were overrunning the front gate. I had nowhere to run and nowhere to hide. I'd be shaking and sweating. My mouth would be dry. Then when I'd finally wake up, I'd check my perimeter, look out all the windows, or go outside to make sure everything was all right. I was always armed, but I never had to use my weapon."

Whiskey blocked out those night terrors, and he stayed drunk for his first couple of weeks back home on Montana's Fort Belknap Indian Reservation. Then his parents got worried about him and checked King into a hospital, where the doctors knocked him out with shots every time he woke up. "I finally decided they were trying to kill me with the shots, so I checked out," he said. "After that, my mom and dad took turns sitting up with me every night for the next couple of months."

In the early '70s, he took off and hit the road. "I was just bumming around on different reservations," he said. "I'd work a little and drink all the time." Somewhere along the line, he found a girlfriend, got her pregnant, married her, and divorced her a couple of years later. "I was always drinking and raising hell."

Then he went to work for the Bureau of Indian Affairs road department at Fort Belknap. It was a job that he worked for 10 hours a day, four days a week. "I'd start drinking on Thursday, all Friday and Saturday, and then taper off on Sunday," he said.

That went on until 1987, when he took a break from the road department to help his uncle and several neighbors with spring calving and branding. Booze was a huge part of that experience. "We'd brand during the day, taking frequent beer breaks, drink into the night, close the bars down, and then come back again the next morning," said King. "Someone had a bottle of brandy that no one wanted so I took it and drank the whole damn thing. The next morning, I was sicker than hell. In fact, I was sick for three straight days, couldn't even keep water down. And after that, I quit drinking. I knew if I didn't quit, it would kill me."

Quitting cold turkey was enormously difficult. With abstinence, the nightmares came back full force. And King didn't think he had any medical benefits because he didn't have an honorable discharge, only a general discharge. "When I left 'Nam, the captain told me he'd see to it that I never got any benefits, that my life would be pretty well screwed up forever," he said.

That's a common military reaction that the Veterans for America (VFA) is still trying to fight today. "A significant number of service members suffering from PTSD and/or mild TBI are simultaneously entering the military justice system," it reported. "This raises the important question of whether it is fair to punish a service member suffering from service-related PTSD and/or TBI for unacceptable behavior when the behavior is symptomatic of a wound that the military has neglected to initially diagnose or treat."

Self-medication for pain

Booze is a common way for vets to numb themselves against the pain they have suffered and still experience, but it's also a good way for the military to get rid of soldiers who are beginning to cause problems. "Without help, people with PTSD turn to drinking and drugs," said the VFA report. "People with traumatic brain injury have discipline and anger issues. And yet unit commanders still say that PTSD and brain injury are not an excuse for bad behavior. VFA is concerned that there is no mechanism for halting or reversing the discharge process once it has been initiated, no matter the mitigating circumstances, nor is there any review of discharges by an entity outside the chain of command."

In the spring of 2007, the National Center for Addiction and Substance Abuse (CASA) explored PTSD in a conference entitled, "Compound Fractures: Substance Abuse and Trauma." Eight years before, I'd worked closely with CASA, its Executive Director Joseph Califano (former head of the Department of Health, Education, and Welfare under President Jimmy Carter), and Vice President Sue Foster as I was writing a yearlong series of stories on alcoholism, and they invited me to join them at the workshop. As always, it was very helpful.

"Substance abuse and trauma feed on each other," said Califano. "Combined with stigma and shame, they make treatment more difficult." Califano said national experts are predicting that PTSD rates for Iraqi and Afghan vets will be as high as or higher than they were for Vietnam vets. "And we know that drug use increased after that war," he added. "Heroin use reached record levels after that war."

"I'm seeing people who don't show problems on the battlefield, but as soon as they begin to experience the 'PTS' part of post-traumatic stress disorder, they begin to dull their senses with drugs," said Colleen A. Matter, staff psychologist at the Rochester, New York, VA Outpatient Clinic.

That's also a new phenomenon, agreed Dr. Paul Arbisi, associate professor and staff clinical psychologist at the VA Medical Center, Minneapolis. "The rapidity with which people are turning to drugs after their return is much more rapid today than it was in the Vietnam era."

Stress is one of the most important factors relating to the use of drugs, said Dr. Nora Volkow, MD, director of the National Institute on Drug Abuse. "Genetics make up about 50 percent of the risk factor, but environmental stress makes up the other half."

Stress can change the way the brain functions, she said. "Both substance abuse and stress collide in dopamine. It is responsible for our ability to receive pleasure, and it motivates our instincts for survival. If you have an animal devoid of dopamine, it will not eat food. And drugs of abuse basically do that. Acute stress can do the same thing as those drugs."

The prefrontal cortex, which is the decision-making part of the brain, regulates the amygdala, which is part of the limbic system, she said. But children and teenagers are less able to control those emotional urges because the pre-frontal cortex undergoes its major development phase while children are in their teens. Remember that the average age of a combat soldier in Vietnam was just 19 years old.

Life on the line

Robert King is another example of a combat vet who came unglued after serious combat. And faced with a choice of medical treatment or discipline, the Army chose punishment, as it usually does. But King's case is a classic scream for help.

King was shipped to Vietnam in December 1968 with an artillery battalion, shelling things no one could see. "Humping ammo," as he puts it. He bounced around without seeing much action until he volunteered to become a radio operator. Then it got hairy.

"My first firefight was kind of spooky," he said. "I was with a Marine lieutenant and a gunnery sergeant (ARVN advisors). We were bouncing around in the jungle and drove right into a North Vietnamese bunker complex. One guy peeked over the edge of the armored personnel carrier, and there was a pop-pop-pop of an AK-47. If I'd poked my head over the edge, I'd have been shot. The sergeant pulled the pin on a grenade, dropped it over the side, and it was done. Then he went out, picked up the AK-47, an ammo belt with a little star on it, and a helmet that had a picture of this guy's girlfriend taped inside it."

So they got instant battlefield souvenirs.

Skirmishes and incoming fire became more frequent as the 2/7 ARVN Armored Cavalry unit shadowed by A Co. of the 1/77 Armored 5th Mechanized Infantry Battalion rolled toward an old Special Forces camp at Long Vei near Khe Sanh and near the Laotian border where they settled in for the night.

"When I woke up, all kinda shit was happening, mortar rounds and small arms fire and explosions. I grabbed my rifle and dove into an old bomb crater, and it jammed up. The lieutenant was screaming and yelling at me to call in fire, but the 40th Artillery got hit at the same time so we couldn't call them in. The 5th Mech did have some tanks in there. You could see NVA [North Vietnamese Army] running through the camp, sometimes 10 feet away, throwing charges at our personnel carrier. And I could see more of them coming, see their flares advancing."

In the confusion, his radio useless and his rifle jammed, there wasn't much King could do. He sat helplessly and watched it all unfold until an AC-130 Gunship II, known as a "Spooky Gunship" or "Puff the Magic Dragon" arrived on the scene.

"It had these Gatling guns going," he said. "They say it can fly over a football field and put a bullet into every square inch of it. The pilot told us to light up our perimeter so he could see where to go. All the time, we were taking mortar rounds and incoming fire for probably four or five hours.

"I just shut down during the attack, focusing on doing my job. Later, I walked around and checked things out. There were dead people everywhere. I looked under a tank, and there was a guy lying on his stomach with his hands under his chin — I thought he was dead until I saw a little flicker of his eyelid and knew he was still alive. The medevac choppers were coming in while the jets were still diving and dropping bombs all around. Then I saw about 10 ARVN that had been captured by the NVA all tied together and stripped to their shorts; I guess they'd been captured."

King pitched in to help get the wounded aboard the medevac helicopters. "I was like a zombie, just picking bodies up. But while we were medevaccing them out, some of the ARVN [Army of the Republic of Viet Nam] troops that didn't want to fight anymore were jumping into the choppers and I was throwing them off. They'd hang on to the skids and I'd pull them off. All this time, we were still under fire, and planes were dropping napalm. I thought I was doing OK until I saw the door gunner on one of the choppers, his eyes big with fear."

Then it was time for the dead. "We were stacking bodies like cordwood. I think we had about 60 of them. I remember an NVA with a [bullet] hole behind his ear. When I turned him over, the whole rest of his head, the brains and everything, was gone. That did something to me, but I just threw his body on the pile."

In the middle of the carnage, a chopper touched down and an official stepped off, a general in a starched uniform, every medal sparkling in its place. It must have been like one of Bill Mauldin's Willie and Joe cartoons during World War II.

"He walked past me with his uniform all neatly pressed," said King. "Right behind him was an aide. He came over and told me I was going to get an AR-15 [disciplinary action] for not saluting the commanding general of I-Corps [the historic Army corps headquartered in Fort Lewis, Washington]. I told him I was stacking those piles of bodies, that we were still under fire from those snipers across the Laotian border, and that if I saluted anyone, the snipers would know that was an officer and take him out. Then I deliberately saluted the aide, and he took off. I never got the AR-15."

Overall, he spent about 18 days in hostile territory, but much of it King still can't remember. Some of the memories have returned with therapy, but some he can't retrieve no matter how hard he tries. He thinks he lost at least 52 hours. "It became one of my obsessions to figure out what happened in those three days. I try to remember, but I still can't."

Memories blocked

Memory loss is common among vets who've been through severe combat. "I can't remember," sounds pretty common, but the memories they can't recall are some of the most stressful of their lives, the memories you'd think would be imprinted on their brains forever.

Researchers first found that rats confronted with stress they couldn't handle lost brain cells in their hippocampus, the memory center. Later, they found that combat vets with PTSD averaged eight percent less volume in their hippocampus than normal. And still later, at least four studies showed decreased volume in the hippocampus of combat vets suffering from PTSD, which could explain some of the verbal memory deficits and perhaps some of the actual memory loss.

Researchers are now investigating whether this hippocampus volume is a result of stress ... or its cause. The studies of twins mentioned earlier — one exposed to trauma and the other not — showed both had reduced hippocampal volume, suggesting reduced size may have been a pre-existing vulnerability for the disorder rather than a consequence of it.

Under "friendly" fire

Three weeks later there was a problem with a Marine gunship that mistook them for the enemy and strafed them. "The lieutenant and the sergeant told us to stay put, lie down, and aim at the helicopter," says King. "And if he opens up again, we'll bring him down. When he came back again and didn't get any return fire, he realized that he'd screwed up and lined out. I was really relieved that we didn't have to bring an American chopper down."

By the end of May 1969, Robert King's unit was back at headquarters in Dong Ha and then at fire base Charlie I, which was defended by the ARVN Army. "On June 7-9, we got a bunch of incoming and some sappers [combat engineers] tried to overrun our fire base. There were 67 or so who got killed. I was in my bunker with my M-16, watching all that fighting on our outer perimeter. I was going to head to the gate, but the sergeant ordered me to stay put. Even though there were a bunch of tracers and shit flying around, we were relatively safe."

But that feeling of helplessness, of being out of control in a situation, is one of the hallmarks of PTSD.

Point of no return

A couple of weeks later, he was in his bunker again, drinking beer, when a trip flare drifted out of the night sky. That's when King snapped. "I shot the hell out of the trip flare and put a couple of rounds through our unit sign. I emptied my clip, but no one was firing back so I stopped. The sergeant came running out, grabbed my rifle, and put me under house arrest."

King ended up in solitary confinement in the Army Stockade at Long Binh Jail, although he said the Marine guards felt he was completely justified in blowing off a little steam. A psychologist concluded that he was competent to stand trial, so he was court-martialed for wrongful discharge of his weapon. After 15 days in the stockade, he was sent back to his unit, but the Army wouldn't give him his rifle back.

"They put me on a shit-burning detail," said King. "Every day, you'd empty the latrines, haul that stuff out in barrels, bring in diesel fuel, throw a match on it, and watch it burn. They told us they didn't want the Vietnamese to use American shit on their fields, so they'd burn it instead."

By this time, King's anger was erupting in serious fighting, and his superiors prohibited the EM clubs from serving him alcohol. He found it anyway, buying it from Marines and Seabees or crawling through a hole in the wire surrounding the hooch in which he was living. Caught buying booze a couple of times, he ended up back in the brig where he remembers accosting a guard who was mistreating fellow prisoners. "I told him these guys had seen more combat in an hour than he would see in his lifetime, and that's why they were there, that's why I was there."

For mouthing off to a guard, King was sent back to solitary confinement. Stuck in an 8-by-8-by-8 box that served as his cell, he was stunned by a race riot that swept through the compound, broke open his cell box, and freed him. "I didn't want to be free. I went back into one of the boxes and hid there, but then the MPs came in and busted it all up," he said. "There were fists and nightsticks, and we were all pretty well beat up. We were placed 'in the hole,' solitary confinement in an even smaller box with only bread and water for two weeks. When our injuries and bruises were healed, we were released. I got a discharge and was sent home."

He was discharged in Oakland, California, in a Class A uniform with no insignia. As he was looking for the bus station to get back to Montana, a local resident took pity on him. "This guy told me never to tell anyone that I'd been in Vietnam. He told me to go down the street to the Williams Hotel and they'd take care of me. I was feeling pretty rough, so I pushed the dresser and the bed against the door, took the blanket and pillow and slept on the floor."

When he got back to Montana, his attitude wasn't good. "After I came out of that riot, I hated everyone. I even hated myself. And after that, people would just leave me alone — it must have been some sort of look on my face that made people want to have nothing to do with me."

Still learning about booze

Nearly a decade ago, I wrote a 12-month series of stories on alcoholism for the Great Falls *Tribune,* a series that won the Pulitzer Prize for explanatory reporting in 2000; it was subsequently published as a book entitled *Alcohol: Cradle to Grave.* At that time, I reported that about 10 percent of all Americans were alcoholics or alcohol-dependent, but that the rate for Montanans was 15 percent. When I asked why those numbers should be so high in a state as beautiful as Montana, I was told that the extraordinarily low population density led to isolation, which in turn could lead to heavy drinking. I was also told the state's hard-drinking cowboy heritage was another cause.

I learned that alcoholism is a medical illness that has a genetic underpinning. That is, you can get a pretty fair idea of your risk of becoming an alcoholic by looking at the rest of your family — the more alcoholics in the family, the higher your risk. But that's only half of the cause. The other half is environmental. Frequently, people tend to block out pain by drinking, and the more pain they experience, the more they drink. Unfortunately, it's a system that's counterproductive. The more people drink, the more they increase their pain. And they find that their bosses, wives, girlfriends, etc., only tend to get madder at them.

For those stories, I followed a number of hard drinkers and recovering alcoholics around, and I remember that several of them had military backgrounds. I now know that combat experience can be a major cause of pain, leading to a heavy reliance on alcohol. But as I was writing those stories, I never made the connection between the high rate of alcoholism and military service. Montana has more veterans per capita than virtually any other state in the nation. As I think about it, I'd be willing to bet that prior military service is a major factor behind our abnormally high alcoholism rate.

Getting sober and clean

It took decades for King to recover, and giving up alcohol was a huge step. Another was the discovery that he wasn't alone with his problems. In 1987, he participated in a *Cursillo* (a course of spiritual renewal or study) in a Catholic church. "And that sort of opened things up for me. I was listening to all the problems people had, all the tragedies they'd lived through, and all of a sudden, the dam burst. I started crying, and I couldn't quit for a long time."

King also discovered after he quit drinking that his discharge didn't affect his medical benefits, so he got help from drug and alcohol counselors at the Vet Center in Billings and a mental health care program at the Northern Montana Hospital in Havre.

But it was expensive to travel hundreds of miles for medical help, "and they didn't pay hardly anything for travel," he said. "It almost wasn't worth going." In fact, for the past 30 years, the VA has paid disabled vets 11 cents a mile to seek medical help. Montana Sen. Jon Tester finally introduced legislation to get the full federal mileage rate for vets.

"A disabled vet who lives in Plentywood [Montana] and has to travel to Montana's only VA hospital, Fort Harrison in Helena, currently gets reimbursed only $55 for the 500-mile trip," said Tester. "Under my bill, the vet going to see his doctor would get the same as a federal employee traveling for work, $242." But the mileage rate was trimmed to 28.5 cents a mile [around $150] in a conference committee. That somewhat improved rate finally took effect in early 2008.

By contrast, VA officials get 48.5 cents per mile — nearly double what the vets get — when they travel.

Slow walk to recovery

King began to hang out with other vets. "They made me walk in a parade at the dedication of the Montana Vietnam Memorial in Missoula. That was really hard for me," he said. "I was sweating and choking."

Then he took advantage of a 90-day residential PTSD program at American Lake. "They'd drag you through everything, reach down your throat, and rip your heart out. They're so good at what they do that you can't lie to them, and they have a lot of Vietnam vets on their staff," he said.

Back on the reservation, it was soothing to be able to work with livestock again. Some people think of horses as just big dogs, but they proved to be therapeutic. "Working with horses just kind of brought me around again," said King.

After going through the program, King made a couple of trips with other former patients to the Vietnam Veterans Memorial in Washington, DC, including a ceremony on Memorial Day to celebrate the 10th anniversary of the memorial. "After I saw the memorial, I thought it would be a good idea to build a memorial at home."

So he started dragging big boulders off Snake Butte on the Fort Belknap Reservation, built a medicine circle 60 feet wide, and put boulders in place for veterans of World Wars I and II, Korea, and Vietnam. Most of it he did alone in the evenings, but kids from the AmeriCorps and tribal construction workers pitched in periodically. "That did a lot for me, to have a memorial for the people who had died," King said. "It took a lot of anxiety off me."

Without booze, the healing begins

With the emotional release, King's anger melted away and he began to heal. He worked as a fire boss, directing Indian fire-fighting teams across the West, which was healthy because it put King in charge of reacting to dangerous situations and gave him responsibility for his men.

Then a couple of years ago, King's combat experience came full circle. He got a letter from a lady he didn't know in Manchester-by-the-Sea, England, opened it, and a dog tag fell out. "I looked at it and everything matched: my name, Social Security number, and military identification number. It really blew me away," he said. He didn't remember losing a dog tag, but it would have been easy to do. "The Marines tied their dog tags on the laces of their boots," he said. "Then when people got blown away, someone would find a boot with a foot in it and know who you were." So going into combat, he began to tie a dog tag to his boot.

Then he read the letter. The woman wrote that she had recently toured Vietnam with her daughter and had run into a villager who had been working in a field and found the dog tag. He had entrusted it to her, asking her to return it to its rightful owner. She had looked King up and sent him the letter, hoping that she'd sent it to the right person.

"It brought a lot of stuff back," he said. "I was down for about a week, thinking about all that stuff." But this time, King didn't hide in a bottle. He dealt with the emotions with the help of his friends, fellow vets, and counselors. And he framed the dog tag and put it in a place of honor on his wall.

Millions still need help

Gen. Barry McCaffrey, former director of the White House Office of National Drug Control Policy for five years under President Bill Clinton, says that, "Sixteen million Americans have chronic substance abuse problems, and only about five million of them have access to treatment, much of it terribly bad."

McCaffrey is frequently in and out of both Iraq and Afghanistan as an advisor and to visit his son, serving with the 82nd Airborne. He estimates that 150,000 U.S. troops are being supported by 130,000 private security contractors, a number larger than the Department of Defense admits.

During the Vietnam era, he said, troops knew to the day when they'd be out of danger, but today the prospect of extension only adds to the stress of the troops fighting abroad. "Right now, we're routinely extending their terms of duty," the retired four-star general said. "And many of the soldiers in Baghdad today are on their third tour of duty. When they come home, they will have seven months at home before they are eligible for deployment again."

McCaffrey said troops in the field have no official access to alcohol or drugs, but get them anyway. He said cocaine has become a problem among troops.

"If a soldier is under constant fire under extreme weather conditions, brutally hot or cold, plus extreme fatigue, perhaps four hours of sleep a night, they will bring that stress home and they will have problems," he said. "We're going to put two million troops through this phenomenon, and many are going to come back physically or emotionally damaged."

Booze seemed the answer

It's called *self-medication*, and it's a way of blocking out bad memories and dulling the senses. While illicit drugs are a problem, alcohol still remains America's drug of choice, largely because it's legal and easy to get. That was particularly true for the Vietnam vets.

"I was an infantry squad leader along the DMZ," said Michael Charter of San Diego, California, director of a vet group he founded called Patriots Choice. "Our job was to get out there and kill people, and that's just what we did. That's also what they did. North Vietnamese soldiers had us pinned down on the hillsides for 10 or 12 hours several times."

Charter was wounded twice in 'Nam. When he returned in 1969, he found a restless wife and a job that hadn't waited for him. "I attempted to pick up where I'd left off, but after about two years, I realized I didn't fit anymore," he said. "All the things that were very important to my friends were meaningless to me. I would think about Vietnam every day. I continued to do quite well at my job, but I started drinking wine every day. My wife would have a glass or two, but I'd have a bottle. After 10 years, I was an alcoholic, but a functional one."

Increasingly, Charter needed to be alone with his thoughts. With good reason, he said, his wife divorced him, so he quickly remarried a woman he met in a bar. "I was drinking a lot, but I didn't know why," he said. "When I didn't drink, I wasn't a very nice person — you wouldn't want to be around me."

Although he was still quite successful as a commodities broker, a job that demanded his full attention, he started to seek help at the VA in 1989, but, instead, walked out in frustration and fear. "It took me becoming no longer functional with a bottle of vodka beside my bed so I could get a drink in the middle of the night and another in the morning when I woke up," Charter said.

Finally in 1998, he went back to the VA for help and founded Patriots Choice to help other vets with PTSD. Being around other vets gives him a sense of security. "The only place I feel safe anymore is when I go on base," he said.

Song for a war hero

My friend Jack Gladstone — an enrolled member of the Blackfeet Tribe and the founder of a program called "Native America Speaks" in Glacier National Park — watched the destruction of a war hero and wrote a chilling ballad about it.

His subject was Ernest DuBray, his father's best friend. DuBray enlisted in 1942 and was assigned to the Army Air Force as a tail gunner aboard a B-17 Flying Fortress over Europe. As the bombers penetrated Nazi Germany, they suffered a 58 percent casualty rate. The average number of missions before a crew was shot down was 14, the required number to fly before being rotated out was 30; DuBray flew 52. "He was shot down twice, once over the English Channel and once behind enemy lines but he managed to escape," said Gladstone. "He came home as the most highly decorated Indian from Montana, but my dad always said he'd blown one fuse too many." DuBray came home with the Distinguished Flying Cross with three oak leaf clusters.

But he also came home so shattered that he could only function with a huge load of alcohol, so Gladstone wrote this ballad about him:

We became men in the skies above the Reich
Bombing daily, the British bombed by night
We were young then, with dreams to go back home
Some were broken, their shadows left to roam.

Through the green grass of 1942,
We enlisted, sacrificing school.
Only God knew when, or if, we would return.
Our duty was freedom to be earned.

Fortresses suspended in the atmosphere,
The earth lay like a dream miles below.
German fighter aces cut our crews in half.
We fell into eternity in droves.
From the sky.

Ha hey Haw-naw hey-naw
Ha ley-ya hay naw, ha hey-la-hey

Missions became memories by the fall of '45.
Peace tasted sweet for those who survived.
Casualties of war were over, but for some,
Streams of nightmares had really just begun.

If we had the chance to live our lives again
We'd find another way to ease the pain.
Sober circles work to keep our demons down.
Our lives could be close to whole again.

Sometimes Eagles have trouble on the ground.
Ha hey haw-naw Hey-naw
Ha ley-ya hey naw, ha hey-la-hey

Sergeant Ernest C. DuBray and this world parted ways
In the water below St. Mary's Lake.
As a warrior ascended, a Native Son went down.
Sometimes Eagles have trouble on the ground.

Let's remember our heroes whose stars have fallen down
Sometimes Eagles have trouble on the ground.

On June 12, 1963, DuBray got drunk, fell off an irrigation ditch bridge into the waters of St. Mary's Canal, and drowned. Six years later, Gladstone's dad decided sobriety was the right step and took it. Not long ago, Gladstone did the same, remembering the two men so fundamental to the formation of his life. "My image of Ernest's ascension is that this eagle was finally liberated from being bound to Earth," he said.

A problem that won't quit

There's little doubt that alcohol has plagued vets since they returned from the first battlefields, but it's been a real problem since the end of World War II. And it remains a serious problem today.

The Army has seen almost a three-fold increase in alcohol-related incidents between 2005 and 2006. And at least 40,000 Iraqi/Afghan vets — 15 percent of all the OIF/OEF vets treated — have received treatment for substance abuse. "These numbers are only the tip of the iceberg," notes the Iraq and Afghanistan Veterans of America. "Many veterans do not turn to the VA for help coping with substance abuse, instead relying on private programs or avoiding treatment altogether."

It should come as no surprise that jumpy combat vets who are prone to nightmares and flashbacks should try to dull their senses with booze. But it's a symptom that the VA should be alert for. The post-deployment assessment forms that Montana National Guardsmen must answer every six months for their first two years after returning from combat specifically ask whether soldiers are drinking on a daily basis ... and how much. That's a question the counselors across the country should be asking, and it's something the VA should be sensitive to.

- 8 -
Flashbacks — videos that won't stop

Behind some of the Faces of Combat are pictures of battles —
flashbacks of combat. The faces we see may look the same as they
did before service, but what the veterans see may be totally
different. In their heads, they may still be seeing a war that their
bodies left behind years before.

Sam Pappas was alarmed when he saw the armored deuce-and-a-half
truck bristling with Panamanian soldiers parked in front of his house on a
quiet suburban street in Great Falls. It was what he'd been afraid of ever
since he returned from combat in Panama in 1989 with a mission to
topple dictator Manuel Noriega and protect the Panama Canal. Since
then, Pappas said he had spent most of his nights patrolling the perimeter
of his home to make sure that the bad guys didn't sneak in and kidnap his

children. During the day, he'd catnap a bit. And now, he'd let his guard down and they were about to attack in broad daylight.

"I ran to the basement to the gun locker, but I couldn't find the key and I was beating on it to get it open," he said. "My daughter was home at the time and called 9-1-1. The cops came and I was in attack mode, but they talked me down and got me to an ambulance and restrained me. Thank God the gun locker was locked or I would have opened up on the ice cream man."

That's called a flashback. The deuce-and-a-half truck that Pappas thought he saw was actually a Schwan's ice cream delivery truck, but the post-traumatic stress in his mind turned it into a kind of a living nightmare. Flashbacks have been described as a video that plays in your mind — you see it, hear it, feel it, smell it — but you can't turn it off.

No one knows exactly what, if anything, triggers these flashbacks. They're completely unpredictable. Sometimes it's a smell or a sound, something that brings back a memory.

Grant Leland, an Iraqi vet who earlier saw combat in Somalia and Bosnia, tells of driving his car down a three-lane urban highway, looking down at what appeared to be a pothole, then looking up again to find himself in the middle of a convoy going up the same dusty road he had patrolled in a Humvee a year before. He said he knew where he really was — he could hear traffic on both sides of him — but he couldn't see where he was going. So he had to slow his car down and stop in the middle of the highway until the flashback passed. But the worst flashback was when Leland lost his sight altogether. "I thought I'd gone blind," he said. "After a while, I could see again. Then I figured out I was having a flashback of a night battle where they were dropping mortars on us and we were firing back. But that was when I realized I really needed to get help."

Sometimes, flashbacks appear for no reason. Pappas's ex-wife Kay Brower was driving him home from Wal-Mart not long ago, "and I saw three PDF [Panamanian Defense Forces]. One of them had a rocket across his back. They were just walking down the sidewalk. I froze and stared at them. I saw them for seven to 10 seconds, and then they just disappeared."

For Pappas, the PDF were the bad guys. "You had to watch out for them because they'd rob you. They shot a Marine on December 18, a guy who was just going out for dinner. I developed a strong animosity against them."

Three or four times a week, Pappas thinks he's re-experiencing the stench of death. "I still get olfactory hallucinations," he said. "I still smell decomposition, burned hair, and cordite. It's the smell of death."

And that brings back memories of helping unload two Mortuary Affairs trucks in Panama. "We unloaded the bodies of probably 100 Panamanians," he said. "As soon as they opened the truck, the smell told me what it was. A lot of the body bags had bones sticking out of them, and I got a lot of body fluids all over me. There was the smell of burned hair everywhere. I couldn't get that smell off me for weeks, but I didn't realize how much it bothered me until I got home and went out to a buddy's ranch where they were branding cattle. Then it all came back and I started dry-heaving."

Pappas shows the ravages of war

Looking at Pappas today will simply break your heart. He's still a big, burly man with the muscles of a weight lifter. His dad was a command sergeant major, the highest enlisted rank. Growing up in Detroit, all he ever wanted to be was a soldier. He got what he dreamed of, and it crippled him. He's got a brace on one knee, and he walks with a cane that wraps around his wrist for extra support. His face twitches, his eyes blink rapidly, and he stutters. "I'm double disabled," he said, "100 percent physical and 100 percent PTSD."

During a 15-year career with the Air Force security forces, Pappas saw combat in Desert Storm, Desert Shield, and Operation Provide Comfort, working with the Kurds in southern Turkey and northern Iraq. But it was Panama that tore him up the worst.

"The first night in Panama, I could hear the bullets shooting through the trees at us. There were green tracers, so we knew they were AKs [AK-47s, a military rifle favored by Communist forces]. It was weird because they [the tracers] would actually bounce off the trees — you could see them ricochet."

He volunteered to do the initial search of the Panama City airport, a dangerous assignment because it had been occupied by the bad guys. "I saw a Ranger go into one of the latrines to check it out and come hauling out of there with a Panamanian shooting a pistol at him," Pappas said. "We threw a frag grenade into the latrine and started shooting through the walls. Then we went through the entire airport, room by room, never knowing if someone was going to be behind a door in the next room."

Later, that terror became almost routine. "There was a constant fear of not knowing if you're going to get shot or not. It's terrifying. Your adrenaline spikes and stays there. I was eight days without sleep once until I started hallucinating."

Worse than anything was the carnage to civilians just a few days before Christmas. "When they rolled the Bradleys [tanks] out, they just ran over cars. I saw a lot of car seats, crushed presents, families and cars crushed and eviscerated. And these people were Christians. They believed in the same things we do. They have Christmas trees and nativity scenes, and they enjoyed Christmas just as much as we do. And then we had to turn around and nail them."

To prove his point, Pappas loans out a video entitled "The Panamanian Deception" by a group called the Empowered Project, which also said that American tanks drove over civilian cars. It shows half a dozen crumpled vehicles and quotes an eyewitness as having seen, "a great number of civilian cars with whole families inside, kids killed, and drivers torn to pieces and crushed by the tanks." And Pappas doesn't doubt for a moment that it's real. "I've seen some of the same stuff that they filmed," he said.

Many vets have bad anniversaries

Since then, Pappas has a lot of trouble handling Christmas. "That's usually when I go into the hospital," he said. Pappas has been through six PTSD treatment programs, and several of them have helped a lot, he said. But seeing Americans killed beside him made him realize that he could die, too. And seeing Panamanian kids killed made Pappas realize that his kids (twin 10-year-old daughters and a pair of older sons and a pair of older daughters) could be killed as well.

So the flashbacks continue to trouble him. He was catnapping on the sofa a few years ago, heard a sound at the door and looked up to see a PDF soldier standing there. Pappas was off the sofa in a heartbeat, went through the screen door, and had the bad guy on his back, screaming to his daughter to get his rifle. She kept saying, "Dad, don't hurt the postman." Pappas searched the guy, found no weapons, and finally realized that the guy was just delivering the mail.

Pappas has been through a lot, and he continues to suffer. He tries not to watch television — after seeing the national news media sugarcoat what Americans did in Panama, he doesn't trust what he perceives as propaganda anymore — but the images coming out of Iraq torment him. "It makes me want to go back over there real bad," he said. "If I weren't so screwed up, I'd be over there in a heartbeat."

Part of it is a sense of responsibility, he said. He's been in combat, and he knows how to take care of his men in a firefight. But part of it, said his former counselor, Tony Rizzo, is that Pappas is chasing after an elusive adrenaline high. And Pappas knows that's true, too. "When you're in combat, shooting your machine gun, you've never been more alive in your life. Every sense — hearing, sight, and smell — is 100 percent plus. It's a massive surge of adrenaline."

He also has some pretty hellish nightmares. "One that keeps reoccurring is being overrun and shooting at them, but it's like they're Nerf bullets. They only go about 10 feet and they drop. In another, I'm being held down and grab my M-16 and put it up to the guy's throat and pull the trigger and nothing happens. Then I look down and there's no magazine in my gun."

But family is where Pappas is most vulnerable, and one nightmare destroys him. "I'm being held back by a bunch of Panamanians and they grab one of my daughters and stick her feet in a fence. She falls backward and is hanging there, upside down. Then they light her hair on fire and start pissing on her. And I can't do anything. When I get that one, I wake up crying."

Doctors are still trying to understand it

There is a medical explanation for nightmares and flashbacks, but it's not very precise. Researchers are still trying to figure out how we dream, for example, and nightmares and flashbacks are a step beyond that. But doctors do know that we have two different sleep patterns. One is called rapid-eye-movement (REM) sleep; it seems to be the deeper sleep, and 25 percent of our sleep is REM. "This is where your dreaming occurs," said Dr. Murray Raskind, a veteran psychiatrist at the VA hospital in Seattle. "But it's also quite unusual because your major muscles are paralyzed and you don't thrash around much." The reason, he told me, is that the brain does not produce its normal supply of adrenaline (or more technically norepinephrine), the hormone that stimulates the body and raises blood pressure when there's a fight-or-flight situation.

In true combat, you need to be at your highest state of alert, and huge norepinephrine levels are triggered to respond to a life or death situation for you and your buddies. After combat, and particularly after repeated attacks, the body either begins producing more norepinephrine or the receptors become more sensitive. "In the nighttime when you're in a combat zone, particularly in guerilla warfare, the enemy finds the odds are more balanced, so you tend to sleep with one eye open. The norepinephrine doesn't shut down at night; it stays active. So there are intrusions in our normal REM sleep. And these adrenaline surges — no one knows how this works — trigger nightmares that are very different. There's no muscle paralysis. People are thrashing around in bed, apparently recreating some very traumatic experiences. They wake up sweaty and anxious and hypervigilant and have to check for signs of danger. Frequently, they don't know whether they're home in bed or back in Iraq."

Raskind told me that he believes the nightmares and flashbacks are pretty much the same. Although flashbacks occur when people are awake, they usually appear when people are more relaxed. And they can be triggered by specific smells. "I believe they're a sort of nightmare that occurs during the day, often when people are catnapping or daydreaming."

He treats nightmares and flashbacks with an old blood pressure medication called prazosin, which works by blocking the norepinephrine effects on the body. "This old drug is the only one of its class that can be taken by mouth and gets into the brain," he said. "A dozen years ago, I started giving it to Vietnam vets and it blocked the adrenaline surges and blocked those nightmares. Within 500 miles of Seattle, about a quarter of the vets with PTSD are prescribed with prazosin. It's cheap, about a nickel a pill, and it's safe because it's been used by millions of old men with enlarged prostates." Raskind said he doesn't see as many patients with flashbacks, but wouldn't hesitate to prescribe prazosin to them as well.

PTSD is contagious within a family

The PTSD that crippled Pappas also destroyed his marriage, and that came as a total surprise to his family. Kay Brower met him in 1994, four years after Pappas had returned home from Panama; she loved him on sight. "That night, his divorce was finalized, and we met in a bar," she said. "I let my guard down, but he was like the perfect man. He was suffering, but he was honest with me. He told me his continual blinking was just something he did when he got nervous."

Her daughter Kate, then a preschooler, was equally enthusiastic. "When mom first decided to marry him, I was so excited because he was such a perfect man. And then one day, it all stopped."

After their marriage, Brower noticed some strange things about her new husband. His body smelled like bleach, and little shards of what appeared to be glass were leaving the skin of his feet. He also had tics, and his joints ached a lot. But she considered him a war hero and lived with those problems for the next four years that he was on active duty.

As his physical condition deteriorated, however, Pappas was forced into disability retirement, said his former wife, now a counselor with Gateway Recovery Center in Great Falls. "When they took away his military status, they took away his identity. That's when he really started to go downhill. He started to drink quite a bit and smoke."

Her husband seemed to be on edge all the time and got progressively angrier, she said. "We fought a lot, and he had anxiety attacks sometimes when he was drinking." She said he was drinking a pint of whiskey and a six-pack of tall-boy beers every night.

"I tried to tell him that he was a wonderful husband and father in addition to being a hero, but depression set in. That [the military] had been his identity. He just gave up and started drinking more."

The depression led to antidepressants and more pills. "He had so many pills," she said. "With the combination of all the pills, he was just a zombie."

Sometimes, but sometimes not. "He had a lot of conflicts," Brower said. "He killed a couple of people, some at close range. And that affected him. We couldn't snap our fingers at home because he said it reminded him of breaking bones."

Pappas slowly became a "ball of anger," said Brower, yelling frequently at the kids for no reason, drinking and incessantly watching violent television programs. "Toward the end, I put a lock on some of the channels to keep him from that stuff."

Pappas' behavior was hard for her daughter Kate. "You couldn't do anything to make him happy," she said. "If he wasn't asleep, he was watching crime shows. When you tried to talk to him about your day at school, he'd snap at you to shut up."

She remembers vividly the day he hallucinated about the Schwan's truck. "He woke up and didn't know what was going on. He told me terrorists were coming and we'd better get out. He was shouting and trembling real bad, so I called the paramedics."

She remembers having friends over, but hiding them in her room because he was always in the living room watching television in his underwear, ready to explode in anger.

"I'd asked a friend over, and we'd gone to a baseball game because I didn't want her there and because he was being so weird," said Kate. "When we got back, my friend had to help me clean up my room. He had thrown a picture of himself that he had given me on the floor and a little glass statue, so there was glass all over the floor and I was crying and my friend was trying to help me."

It all came to a head on a night Brower said her husband lost it. "He had pulled a gun on me in front of the kids a couple of times and threatened to kill himself," she said. "Then one night in the kitchen, he grabbed Kate by the throat and pulled a knife on me. That was it."

She deliberately took a vacation with the kids, she said, and called him from 1,400 miles away to tell him that she was leaving him. Then she gave him two weeks to calm down before they returned,

Something to be concerned about

There's an object lesson here for all of us. As our troops come home, these scenarios will become more and more common. We need to realize that we're likely to encounter some bizarre behavior as returning vets experience flashbacks in public places. And it points to an increasing need for our police officers to receive training in how to deal with such situations.

- 9 -
America's homeless vets

Faces of Combat sometimes appear looking out from abandoned buildings or from under bridges. There are over 150,000 veterans who will be homeless tonight — some who can't find shelter and some who choose to live on their own, away from others.

A decade ago, a Vietnam vet named Rick Salyer told the Montana National Guard that hundreds of former soldiers were hiding out in solitary camps tucked away in the mountains of Montana, unable to deal with civilian society or still afraid of a phantom enemy that could destroy them. Skeptical, the Guard agreed to sponsor an exercise called Operation Stand Down, which would encourage the vets to come in to the military base at Fort Harrison and begin receiving the help they needed and deserved.

"That first year, we had over 300 homeless vets, none of whom were on the rolls of any of the social services," said Salyer. "Most people think of the homeless as living under bushes and in boxes and under bridges, but these guys had all been living out in the woods."

The National Alliance to End Homelessness estimates that 750,000 to 800,000 people are homeless in America at any given time, and that more than 320,000 of them lack shelter. Reasons range from PTSD to other mental illnesses, substance abuse, and spousal abuse. The majority of the homelessness is urban, the alliance said, but up to 10 percent of it may be rural. "Many rural homeless people live in places we do not see; they are often sleeping in the woods, campgrounds, cars, abandoned farm buildings, or other places not intended for human habitation," it said.

In Montana, the Stand Downs have been continuing, but the numbers have decreased in the past few years because a lot of the vets are getting their claims processed and moving into transitional housing. "If you look at the low-income housing that's been built over the past few years, a lot of them have been filled by veterans," Salyer said.

Salyer said that government housing works for some vets with PTSD; but it just doesn't work for *him*. He, personally, was homeless at the time and remains so today.

Salyer served in 'Nam in 1971-72. "I was a flight engineer/crew chief of a Super C Chinook," he said. "We did five to 10 flight missions a day. Our primary mission was insertion and extraction, and our secondary mission I can't talk about. I saw dead bodies, I saw people get killed, and I picked up dead people. I dealt with the refugee situation on I-corps, and I dealt with mortars 24-7."

His voice trails off there. Asked if he wants to get any more specific, he said only, "No."

Coming home was hard. He was assigned to an aircraft maintenance company in Fort Lewis, Washington, and immediately had issues. "Because their maintenance was sub to what I was used to, I immediately had authority problems. I couldn't accept it. I'd watched in 'Nam, an aircraft go down and kill 33 people."

Disgusted, he left the service in 1977. He tried to go back to college, but found that he couldn't handle what he termed "clueless youngsters" who weren't as intent as he was. Then a professor suggested he take an incomplete to finish up some of his class work. "I did, and the VA sent me a bill for past services due," he said. "And that put me right out on the street.

"I went into the hills," Salyer said. "That's been my escape to keep from being violent or doing something stupid. I used to camp about 17 miles from where my mother lived in the Bitterroot (Mountains). I used to hike in on Christmas day to find a pay phone in Darby to call my mother and wish her a merry Christmas. But I couldn't face my mother because I'd broken every moral rule I'd ever been taught as a Catholic or a Boy Scout. Sometimes I'd come out and work for a rancher or a construction job to get the money to buy supplies. Then I'd load up, get a ride to the edge of road, and walk in with 75 pounds of canned goods on my back. I'd just walk in and out until all my goods were back in camp."

On one of his forays into so-called civilization to earn money, he was set up with a blind date. "I was carrying a heavy load of lust at the time, so I married her," he said. But the marriage didn't last long. "We were married about three years, but I was only there about six months of it," Salyer said. "I'd tell her I was going fishing, and I'd be gone for three months."

Living with Salyer must not have been easy. "I still sleep in a mummy bag that I don't zip up so I can get out of it. If I sleep in a bed, I end up thrashing around in the bed and getting all tangled up in the sheets and blankets until I'm all wrapped up like a mummy. And that's terrifying. My wife used to tell me I was running myself to death, that my feet were going a hundred miles an hour."

So he's been spending most of his time in two camps, one a summer camp and the other designed to minimize the brutal Montana winters. "I have relatives that live up in the Bitterroot Valley, cousins that have packhorses, so I took a miniature cook stove in to my camp there. I have a cave with a hole in the top of it. I put a stovepipe out the top and put a cabin front on it. I have 800 to 1,000 square feet of living space. I also have a camp near Cascadia, Oregon, that's on a guy's property. I have a root cellar there where all my stuff is stored. I come in with 16-by-20 tarps and make a house out of it. In Cascadia, I'm about four miles from the nearest person who I only see once a year when I tell them I'm going in. In the Bitterroot, I'm about 12 miles off the highway. I stay there three to six months."

But the past couple of Montana winters have been a little hard on a vet facing retirement age, even though Salyer looks like an aging hippie in sandals with his graying hair neatly tied back in a ponytail. "The last three years, I've been going down south to the desert. The year before, I spent November to March up near Park Lake, but it was just too hard on my body so a guy came in on a snowmobile and brought me out."

Why does Salyer do this to himself? "I've been in therapy for 13 years now trying to figure that out. I just don't put up with people. I'm not into conflict or gossip or TV. I'm just not social."

Over the years, he's found that doctors and medications have either been ineffective or have made his situation worse. However, the aforementioned prazosin helps him function during the days. "But I can't take it at night. If I do, I don't wake up through the nightmares and I beat myself to death, running and screaming. It's good I'm out in the woods so people don't have to listen to me."

But he has been trying to help other vets through a program called "Vet-to-Vet," which pairs the older vets up with the disabled kids from Iraq and Afghanistan. It seems to help both. "My saving grace has been the Vet-to-Vet support group, so I've been working with them," Salyer said. "It does me a lot of good to help people, but there's no healing in me. It gives me the opportunity to socialize, but that's about all. This is all the life I'm going to get."

Not much help for homeless vets

The VA estimates that on any given night, there are approximately 154,000 homeless vets, but twice that many experience homelessness at some point during any given year. The majority of these vets served in Vietnam; 96 percent are male, and 45 percent of them suffer from mental illness, including PTSD.

Mental illness is a touchy subject with most vets because they believe that labeling them with a pre-existing mental illness is just a way the government avoids responsibility. "If they tag the bipolar on them, they only have to pay them a reduced amount for PTSD. By telling them they're bipolar or have substance abuse or relationship issues, they avoid the PTSD issue. This is our government screwing us," maintained Salyer.

And even the help that's available to vets without mental health issues is insufficient. There's a VA program for the homeless called the Homeless Providers Grant and Per Diem Program that provides funding to community-based, faith-based, and public organizations offering transitional housing for vets. But the maximum daily rate of $31.30 per vet is far less than the cost of providing service in most parts of the country.

"It is my belief that the goal of the VA should be to not only provide veterans with a bed for the night and a meal, but to provide them with the resources that they need to obtain permanent housing, a steady job, and a renewed sense of self worth," said Rep. Michael H. Michaud, D-Maine, chairman of the House Veterans Affairs Health Subcommittee.

But America is nowhere close to that goal. "The tragedy of homeless veterans is that we know what we need to do to prevent it, but neither the military nor the VA bureaucracy is ready to do this," said Rep. Bob Filner, D-California, chairman of the House Committee on Veterans' Affairs. "We also know the repercussions of not doing something. The military should insist on mandatory screening when troops are discharged, and the VA must be prepared to provide comprehensive services."

Increasingly, that outreach must also be provided to women.

"VA and its providers are also grappling with how to accommodate the needs of the changing, homeless veteran population that will include increasing numbers of women and veterans with dependents," said Daniel Bertoni of the Government Accounting Office.

"While the vast majority of homeless veterans are male, female veterans are the fastest growing segment of this population," Michaud said. "Women homeless veterans face similar challenges to their male counterparts, but they are very likely to have experienced serious trauma, including abuse or rape, and a significant number have children to support. VA programs must be flexible to meet these new challenges."

In the spring of 2008, new VA secretary James Peake and Housing and Urban Development (HUD) secretary Roy Bernadi announced a new $75 million program to provide housing for 10,000 homeless vets nationwide. Broken down by state, it would help 35 vets in Montana. That's a nice gesture, but it doesn't come close to addressing the real need. And again, homelessness is simply a symptom of the problem — just like drinking too much. To be effective, the VA must deal with the reasons why the vet can't take care of himself.

Safe housing for the short term

A number of cities have opened transitional housing for homeless vets. In Helena, the Montana Veterans' Foundation opened the Willis Cruse Home as a transitional facility. It currently has beds for 11 vets and a resident manager. Vets can stay up to two years, as long as they obey certain rules, including staying free of alcohol and drugs. There's also a curfew they must observe.

A brick storefront building on a residential street, it now features three large bedrooms, a communal kitchen, a living area with overstuffed chairs, and a computer nook where residents have Internet access and word-processing equipment to print out their résumés.

"I was the first resident through their doors," said manager Rick Nicholson. "And I liked it so well I just stayed on. I have my own apartment in a separate building, just behind this one."

Although it was an adjustment at first, the neighbors have accepted the Cruse Home, said case manager Lucinda Leon, a slender blonde who solicits donations to run marathons and donates them for group home expenses. "When we first came here, there was some opposition in the neighborhood, but now they're our biggest supporters," she said.

"That's because we set rules and enforce them," added Nicholson.

Calling all vets who need supplies and services

A light rain was falling in Great Falls on a Saturday morning as vets groups and the VA launched the city's first Stand Down at the Montana ExpoPark. Organizers were buoyed by the fact that they'd served about 125 vets, most of them homeless or close to destitute, in their first four hours Friday afternoon.

Rick De Blasio, a homeless coordinator for the VA in Denver, was on hand to help out. A former street outreach coordinator, he's been involved with Stand Downs across the Northwest.

"This is the VA's 20th year of reaching out to homeless vets and providing them with shelter and services," he said. In the beginning, the VA estimated there were 250,000 homeless vets who needed help, but persistent outreach has dropped that number to about 195,000. "We've made a dent, but we still have a long way to go," he added.

"The VA has been changing its theory on why so many vets are homeless," said De Blasio. "We used to think that most of it was due to combat exposure. But this isn't strictly due to combat stress. There's a percentage of that, but most have mental health or substance abuse problems that have gone untreated. Many soldiers come into the service with these problems to begin with, and those worsen when they leave a highly structured environment. More than 70 percent of the vets we see on the streets have mental health or substance abuse problems."

While some of the homeless vets live in camps or hide out in sheltered areas that the public seldom sees — abandoned buildings or under bridges — most of them float from place to place, doubling up or tripling up with other vets who've found temporary housing, said De Blasio. "Most of them just blend in with other homeless folks. They keep to themselves and keep their military service private."

Across the gym-sized room at the ExpoPark, there's a pile of military surplus gear being given away in duffle bags, and a number of vets were walking out laden with free clothing. "A lot of the vets don't want to go back into camo fatigues," notes De Blasio. "They say they've already had too much of that."

Still, he has no doubt the Stand Down was serving those it was intended for. "I've talked with a lot of people, and I'm confident that most of them are vets," he said. "And I've been impressed with how many of them are taking advantage of the VA system."

Medics were giving free blood pressure and vision checkups, and a barber was providing free haircuts. Lori Pike of the Center for Mental Health provided about a dozen PTSD evaluations, but mostly made referrals and listened to peoples' stories.

"Not long ago, we had a vet who was living under a bridge," said Pike. "We loaded him up with stuff and sent him away happy, but we also gave him a card and asked him to call us. He needs a case manager to get his paperwork started."

A Vietnam vet who couldn't tell his mom what he had done

While some of the vets were in true need, others had already been through their personal wringers and were just there to socialize. That was the case with Jack Jager, a slender Vietnam vet who had always wanted to be a soldier and joined the Army straight out of high school. Jager, a truck driver now, has been sober for the past 11 years and tries to laugh his way through most of his pain. But as Rodger McConnell, one of the Stand Down organizers, notes, "He wears the face."

Jager says he is an alcoholic, married four times, and thought it was normal. "Ten years after Vietnam, I didn't have a clue. Reality to me was war, and everything else was an illusion. You accept your fate, which is to die, and then when you don't die, you don't know what to do with your life."

He was a scout dog handler, protecting the perimeters for the 173rd Airborne. That meant he lived in the field for the most part, using his dogs like bird dogs to flush out enemy soldiers or to sniff out mines and booby traps. That put him on the cutting edge of combat.

"We got overrun once, and that was my last combat experience," he said. "We ran into a camp of NVA regulars, and our battalion commander told us to withdraw a little; but in the evening we got surrounded. Later, I found out it was called the Easter Massacre because it happened on Easter Sunday. Out of the 21 men in our squad, we had 11 killed and six wounded. I remember a guy with his arm blown off asking how the hell he could load his rifle with just one hand. So we withdrew. We had a river at our backs, and two guys who were mortally wounded tried to do their best to hold them off. We slipped into the river, floated downstream, got out on the riverbank, and spent most of the day eluding them."

When he got back to Montana, he said he was able to hold down a job at first, but he was nervous about living in a house. He found a wooded area behind his apartment, built a camp, and lived there with his dogs for company and protection. His breaking point came when his mother looked him in the eye and said, "Jack, what happened to you?" And that was a question he just couldn't answer.

"I felt very guilty," he says. "There are things I did that I felt very guilty about. I was brought up right, brought up to do right, but in war, the compassion is not there. Human beings were not made to kill each other. I saw some soldiers who just could not pull the trigger on an adversary face to face, and they died. After all the depravity of war was over, I was afraid people would know what I was, so I just ran away from it."

Stand Down winds down

By the time the Stand Down was completed, organizers estimated they served about 250 vets and between 350-400 people, including family members. They had two semi-truckloads of surplus gear, roughly 63,000 pounds, and gave away about 35,000 pounds of it — duffle bags full of fatigue pants and shirts, socks, and underwear, raingear and overcoats. "We had a lot of blankets, including some that were still in their original containers," McConnell said. "And we gave away 300 or 400 extra-cold-weather sleeping bags that were really quite nice and quite expensive."

The blood pressure, dental evaluations, and vision check stations remained busy all day, he said. "And a hearing specialist volunteered to come if we could get him a quiet place to do his exams. McCollum RVs was kind enough to lend us an RV, and we set it up outside. It stayed busy all day."

Still lives a military life

Mel, a vet who's been living under a bridge for the past eight years, decided to not go to the Stand Down because it was too wet to bother walking a mile to Montana ExpoPark that Saturday morning. Instead, one of the organizers, Don Scott, brought him a care package to the Town Pump mini-mart where he regularly stops for coffee.

"I stopped in Saturday morning and found a big bundle waiting for me," said Mel, a 64-year-old with a bushy salt-and-pepper beard and cautious eyes that weighed me, a relatively well-dressed stranger joining him for a cup of coffee. A field jacket was too small for him, he said, but he had cold-weather gear anyway. He valued the extra-cold sleeping bag, but already sleeps in one just like it and has two intermediate bags besides. "When it gets real cold, I can stuff one of the intermediates in the cold-weather bag and it'll take me down to about 60 below," he said. "And my dog sleeps with me, sometimes almost on top of me."

As Mel sips his coffee and talks, his dog Sarah sleeps on a blanket outside the store. One of the store employees refers to the Dalmatian as the store mascot. Cashiers smoking their cigarettes outside the store regularly talk to her without expecting an answer. It's a great place for a homeless vet to almost live because it not only has restrooms to wash up in, but it has a coin laundry where he can keep his clothes clean.

Mel enlisted in the Army in 1961 and was stationed along the East German border. "I was in a forward operating post when [President John F.] Kennedy was shot," he said. "It was a pretty tense time. When you heard a noise, you shot. But it's not like the spray-and-pray (automatic) weapons today. It was one-shot, one-kill back then."

When Mel was leaving the Army, he was urged to re-enlist and serve in Vietnam. As an inducement, he was allowed to test-fire the brand-new M-16. "I put a 20-round magazine in it, and it jammed seven times on me," he said. "There was all sorts of brass hanging around, and I told 'em, 'I'm not going into combat with that piece of crap. You give me your little speech, I'll sign that I heard it, and then I'm walking.'"

He left the Army and spent the next couple of decades working odd jobs in Montana and Wyoming, ranching and also working sometimes as a security guard. "But as I got older, I found I had a lower and lower tolerance for BS. There are a lot of people walking around and making themselves look self-important, talking on their cell phones all the time. I didn't want any part of them any more."

In those first couple of decades, he hid out in a bottle. "I was a solitary drinker," he said. "When I was drinking, I wanted to be alone. But I figure I paid for the Cadillacs of a lot of bartenders."

About two decades ago, he quit drinking. "I woke up one morning, went to wash my face, and didn't recognize the face looking back at me," Mel said. "So I quit and haven't had a drink since."

He worked for the Rescue Mission for a while, and then began looking for a place where he could camp out. "I was getting sick of the way things were going," he explained. "We should never have been in

Vietnam — no reason to fight for people who won't fight for themselves — and I feel the same way about Iraq."

A couple of cops recommended a secluded spot under a local bridge. "They knew I didn't drink or do drugs, and they knew I wouldn't be a bother to anyone," he said. "They inspected my gear and figured I wasn't going to turn into a Popsicle. They still come by and check on me every once in a while."

Employees at the Town Pump chat with Mel as he sits, killing time on another rainy morning. One of them slips him a bag of hot dogs that had been roasting too long and would have been thrown away. "If the sandwiches don't sell, they'll bag 'em up for me and we'll take them back to camp and eat them."

Mel and Sarah live in a one-man/one-dog pup tent on the banks of the Missouri River. It's lashed to a couple of tree branches to keep it from blowing away in high wind, and it's stuffed with sleeping bags that Mel sleeps on top of during warm weather or burrows beneath when the weather gets colder. In the brush, he has a stool to sit on when he reads (when it's warm and light) as well as a little fire pit in the gravel of the riverbank a few feet away. His camp is almost invisible; there's a road about 10 yards above him, a river a few feet below him, and a big concrete interstate bridge shields him from above. His camp is about half a mile from my newspaper office, and he'd been living there for years without my knowing it, which made me feel fairly stupid.

When I visited Mel's camp early in the fall, he was constantly alert for a kitten hiding out on the hillside and watching intently. Someone had dumped the kitten, only a few months old, and it had been hanging around and sneaking down to the camp to steal food whenever it could. So Mel was feeding it, gradually taming it.

A couple of months later as we were having coffee together in the mini-mart, Mel announced, "We've got a new addition to our family." It turned out the kitten had slipped into his tent right before the first snowfall. "It burrowed right down in the sleeping bag with me, and I had to be real careful when I turned over that I didn't crush it," he said. "Then after a couple of nights, it lay down by Sarah. I told her to relax and let the little bugger be, and she did. I think the little guy's gonna work out just fine."

By Christmas, Mel had named the kitten Lil Bit "because I could pick him up in my hand and he only weighed a lil bit." A ball of energy, Lil Bit kept Mel amused. "He crawls out on one of the branches above my tent, drops down, and uses the tent as a slide," he chuckled. Through the holidays, folks have been slipping Mel money and wishing him a merry Christmas. He figures he ended up with about $85 in presents. "And the girls down here fixed me a real nice chicken dinner," he said. "We had a real good Christmas."

About the only people who ever see him at home are fishermen and the people floating down the river, and Mel generally chats with them. Sarah alerts Mel when she hears foot traffic on the bridge or anyone messing around in their area. About a decade ago, a transient was beaten to death in that same general area, but Mel doesn't seem worried because he stays on guard most of the time.

During the day, Sarah accompanies him as Mel picks up aluminum cans from curbs and dumpsters. For years, I've picked up cans just because they're an eyesore that should be recycled, but now I wait until I've got a stash in the back of my pickup truck and drop them off with Mel, although he really doesn't need the help anyway. He said he works three or four hours a day and averages about $300 a month. "You'd be amazed at the stuff I find that people have thrown away," Mel said. "I could have a whole bandoleer of cell phones. And the funny thing is that most of them work."

About six weeks before, he found a couple of .22 rifles in a dumpster. "I took them down to the police station," he said. "I figured they didn't belong there."

He also finds a lot of books, many not worth bothering about but a few that are worth reading. He's fascinated by military history, and is reading some military fiction by an author whom Mel believes borrows quite a bit from other authors. "I think that's called plagiarism," he observed, dryly. Although most of his conversation is about military matters, he said his pup tent lifestyle isn't necessarily an attempt to relive his service experience.

So far, collecting and selling aluminum cans is his sole source of income. But Mel said it's enough to feed him. "I have no rent, no utilities, and no bills," he explained. Next year, he plans to apply for Social Security, "but I see no reason to change my lifestyle," he said.

Asked about his combat experience, Mel said he was never really in combat, and he doesn't believe he has PTSD. But he's clearly obsessed with the military, and that didn't make sense to me. Later, I questioned Joe Underkofler, director of the VA Health Care Services in Fort Harrison outside Helena. "I've worked with vets for 30 years," he said. "And I've found that the military experience can become a highlight of a vet's life. It's when they felt the most fulfilled, the most needed, and the most disciplined and focused. It's very much like a high school football player who keeps his trophies in his trophy room. For a number of vets, that military experience is a remembrance of the most important time of their lives."

- 10 -
Occupation: pushing papers

Faces of Combat can be seen pressed up against the windows of the health care system — hungry for help and desperate to get inside. The doors are sometimes so tightly sealed (usually with red tape) that deserving vets can't get in. Some give up. Some keep working until justice is done.

"If you don't give your life to the military, you give it to the VA," said Kevin Vernon, a fourth-generation vet who survived Operation Desert Shield/Desert Storm, but who is not sure he'll be able to outlive or outlast the VA. He's been battling the bureaucrats now for a dozen years and has come to realize that's he's seriously outnumbered. It takes up so much of his time that it has become like a fulltime job. In fact, you could say that Vernon's main line of work these days is fighting the VA.

When Vernon came back from the Persian Gulf War, he didn't think he was disabled. "No one made me aware I had a problem," he said.

"They gave us a questionnaire with about 10 boxes," and he answered them to the best of his ability ... at that time. He answered yes to feelings of fatigue, adding that he was always feeling run down. He answered yes to having recurring thoughts about his experience in Desert Storm/Desert Shield. But, in fairness to the VA, he denied having nightmares or trouble sleeping.

It may have been that the nightmares came later, but to be honest, Vernon just wasn't thinking very clearly. "I don't remember my first year back because I was drunk most of it," he said.

His wife recognized the danger signs, including a husband who was incredibly on edge all the time. "I don't even sleep in the same bed with my wife anymore," said Vernon. "I'm afraid I'm going to hurt her if she touches me during the night and startles me."

Finally, his wife convinced him to seek private counseling in Great Falls, which he did from 1992-93. His counselor suggested he file a claim with the VA, and that's where the whole thing started.

In 1993, Vernon went to Montana's VA center at Fort Harrison for a mental health evaluation. "The shrink put me on trazodone [an antidepressant] and told me to be on my way. He told me to take half a pill before going to bed. If that didn't work, take a whole pill. And if that didn't work, take a pill and a half." But the medication was apparently just a stopgap because the VA wasn't sure what to do with Vernon. "They diagnosed me with PTSD, but they couldn't give me a rating because they said they had no proof of a stressor," Vernon said.

That decision came January 21, 1995. The VA said: "Military discharge certificate (DD Form 214) shows the veteran received the Southwest Asia Service Medal. Primary specialty was fighting vehicle infantryman. No specific combat ribbons were issued. In his statement dated August 29, 1993, the veteran cites numerous combat related stressors. On the VA mental status exam, a diagnosis of post-traumatic stress disorder was made. In order for a service connection to be granted for PTSD, there must be a medical evidence of PTSD and a recognizable, verifiable stressor. Rating as to service connection is deferred pending response from the Department of the Army regarding claimed stressors."

By July 16, 1996, there was no evidence that Vernon had been stressed, so the VA denied his claim for PTSD. It said: "In order to provide further research concerning specific combat incidents and casualties, Mr. Vernon must provide the most specific date possible, location of the incident, numbers and full names of casualties, unit designations to the company level, and other units involved. The PTSD unit can verify only specific combat incidents as recalled by Mr. Vernon. In order to conduct meaningful research, he must provide the 'who, what, when, and where' of each stressor. The veteran has not provided such information to date."

Vernon said he doesn't understand why the VA didn't know these things already, based on his unit designation and what it had been through, but he did his best to lay it all out for them.

A world of death

Vernon was a gunner on an M2 Bradley fighting vehicle. Don't be confused by the term "vehicle" — the Bradley is a tank, with a $3.2 million price tag. It's a 33-ton armored tank that holds a crew of three (a commander, gunner, and driver) as well as six fully equipped infantry soldiers. Its main weapon is a 22mm M242 Bushmaster chain gun, basically a small cannon, that fires up to 200 rounds per minute. It can change ammunition at the flick of a switch from a high-explosive incendiary round with tracers to an armor-piercing discarding sabot, which proved to be capable of knocking out most Iraqi vehicles, as well as some T-55 tanks. The Bradley also carries a pair of TOW2B computer-guided missiles capable of destroying hostile tanks at up to 2.3 miles. In addition to the chain gun, the Bradley has an M240C machine gun with 2,200 rounds of 7.62mm ammunition. Packed with firepower and equipped with heat-sensing radar capable of identifying a human being solely by temperature, the Bradley is highly maneuverable with speeds up to 41 mph.

Vernon said his unit moved into Iraq on February 22, 1991, two days ahead of the general invasion, to open the way for VII Corps to roll through. And those first two days were relatively uneventful, all the way up to the second night in Iraq. "Then we started getting mortars — whump, whump, whump — in the middle of a dust storm," said Vernon. "After the mortar attack, we went a little further and ran into people walking in the middle of the desert in a diamond formation. When we were given the order to engage, I went to my main gun. It was like lobbing grenades at people. Two shots and they just disappeared. After that, all our training just kicked in. We went up a berm to a trench where more guys were shooting small arms at us. We were told weapons free, which means 'When in doubt, take 'em out.' But they were so well entrenched that we couldn't get a shot at them, so I put the barrel of my gun straight up in the air and blasted shells down on them. That took them out. Another hour or two further, we found an ammo truck and a howitzer with no one around them except some guys in a dune buggy with guns and explosives. We took them out, too." Since no one wanted the howitzer to be useful to the enemy, Vernon said he switched to armor-piercing shells and destroyed a lot of abandoned equipment.

Then it was like a mirage, a guy with a briefcase walking through the desert. They ordered him to surrender, but he declined. So they tried to take him out, but never could manage to hit him. Finally, they gave up and left him to another unit. As they rolled under an overpass, Vernon saw movements out of the corner of his eye, so he waved his gun barrel toward the edge where the bridge met the road. He didn't want to fire because he didn't want to bring the overpass down on his Bradley; as he hesitated, a family scuttled out and ran for better shelter.

Finally, his unit reached a major intersection somewhere along Highway 8 and took up a position right in the middle of the road. "I probably had 250 kills right there," he said. "When the Iraqi trucks came down the road, I'd shoot out the engine block. Each truck held about 20 people, and when they jumped out, I'd put a round on one side of the truck and then a round on the other. You'd think someone would tell them to go a different way, but they just kept coming. Once while I was reloading, I got a call, 'Verndog, you've got a truck coming right at you.' I swung my barrel around just as the truck was streaking past me. Right then, my buddy Tucker shot at that truck right over my back deck. The truck blew up, and it was just full of troops. His shot probably saved our lives."

But it wasn't just soldiers out there in the desert in the middle of the night. "We saw a vehicle coming down the road that appeared to have a tripod in front of it, maybe some kind of a gun mount. I asked the lieutenant, and he said it *looked* like a gun mount — take it out. I put a shot through the engine block, and a whole family jumped out and ran into the desert. I thought, 'Good, glad you made it.'

"And there was another old guy, sitting on an overpass rocking. We didn't pay that much attention to him because he seemed pretty harmless. Suddenly he stood up, and his guts fell out. That really got to me, that and the sight of another guy running for safety on the nubs of his legs."

The other thing that got to Vernon was looking at the carnage the next day. "When we went by, we could see a guy slumped over the wheel of his car with gray matter where his head should have been. Destroyed cars with women and kids in them. There were a lot of dead people where they shouldn't have been."

VA needs more proof

By July 22, 1997, it became obvious the VA wasn't buying the stressors he had described.

"Service connection for post-traumatic stress disorder requires medical evidence establishing a clear diagnosis of the condition, credible supporting evidence that the claimed inservice stressor actually occurred, and a link, established by medical evidence, between symptomatology and the claimed inservice stressor," it wrote.

"If the claimed stressor is related to combat, service department evidence that the veteran engaged in combat or that the veteran was awarded the Purple Heart, Combat Infantryman Badge, or similar combat citation will be accepted in the absence of evidence to the contrary as conclusive evidence of the claimed inservice stressor. Additionally, confirmed prisoner of war status is considered conclusive evidence of the claimed inservice stressor. The evidence available for review does not establish that a stressful experience sufficient to cause post-traumatic stress disorder actually occurred."

And yet the post-traumatic stress was clearly there. "I couldn't sleep without a gun," he said. "To this day, I have to have it within arm's reach. I had nightmares, cold sweats, and a lot of hostility toward people. I kept seeing the dead kids and women in my nightmares. And then when

I woke up, I'd be back in the desert again — I could feel the wind and the openness, even though I was sleeping in a closet."

His only physical injury, ironically enough, came as his unit was unloading gear off a flatbed truck right before the Gulf War. Vernon was hit by a loaded duffel bag. The lock ripped his scalp, and the weight of the bag slammed him down onto an ammo case, jamming the joints of his jaw up into his skull. He was bleeding pretty freely so he got his scalp stitched up; however, the injury to his jaw got progressively worse over the years.

After he got out, he spent a couple of years trying to get disability benefits. Fighting the VA began to seem futile to Vernon, so for about eight years, he gave up. "I remember calling the VA and getting transferred 11 times before I ended up with the same woman I'd started with. It's incredibly frustrating to deal with the VA," he said.

So he used some of his GI benefits to go back to school at DeVry Tech in Phoenix and got a job with Intel in Albuquerque as an electrical technician. He stayed there for eight years, in part because Intel put him in an emergency response unit that kept his adrenaline level up. That kept him from getting bored. But his helmet began irritating his head injuries, causing an increasingly severe series of headaches that finally forced him to quit.

Taking on the challenge

With limited prospects in New Mexico, Vernon came back to Montana where his dad, a vet who had served two tours in Vietnam, informed him that he couldn't win against the VA. That was all the challenge Vernon needed. "I'm the son of a 'Nam vet, and there was no love between my father and me. He was distant and cold. For the longest time, I didn't understand it. Then I went into combat myself, and it was like a light bulb turned on."

So he set out to prove that his dad was wrong. His first step was to prove the Army had screwed up on his combat medals. On January 20, 2005, the Army conceded that he was actually due the Combat Infantryman Badge and the Kuwait Liberation Badge. So fourteen years after the fact, it awarded both to him.

That changed the whole equation. On August 25, 2005, the VA awarded Vernon a 30 percent disability for PTSD, 20 percent disability for temporomandibular joint syndrome (TMJ), and another 10 percent for cervical myositis.

Vernon felt he deserved more so he appealed, particularly for the TMJ. "Right now as it stands, I have to take ibuprofen 800 mg three times a day, hydrocodone 750/500 three times a day, Valium 2 mg three times a day, and Prozac 20 mg one time a day. This medical regimen is the only thing that keeps me from committing suicide from the pain. I know the doctors would not prescribe those medications if it was not beneficial to me. I don't understand why the VA does not understand this and how much pain I go through," he wrote on March 1, 2006.

Five days later, the VA told Vernon that he was 80th on a list of appeals that a Board of Veterans Appeals would hear in Fort Harrison, but that it was unlikely the board would be able to hear more than 40 appeals that year.

On May 5, 2006, Vernon responded: "This condition [TMJ] has caused me to not be able to work and have to work only part time, about two hours a day due to the pain which at most times is unbearable and I cannot concentrate on my job functions and also due to the medications that I have to take to keep the pain under control makes me incoherent, drowsy, and not able to function as a husband, father, and employee. On April 19, 2006, I was taken to the emergency room at Benefis Hospital for severe pain to my right jaw joint and pain to my right ear. I was given two shots of adivant, one shot of Toradol, and one shot of morphine to control the inflammation and pain. The cause of the pain was eating a simple turkey sandwich on normal white bread. While eating my jaw made a loud pop and instantly I had uncontrollable pain in my jaw and my head. Ten minutes later was when my ear started to hurt and that's when the decision was made to go to the emergency room."

On June 28, 2006, the VA said his appeal would be delayed. "We are still working on your request for an in-person hearing at the Ft. Harrison Regional Office before a member of the Board of Veterans' Appeals from Washington, DC. Unfortunately, we were unable to include your appeal on the docket for the Travel Board hearings that recently concluded. We expect it will be another 10-14 months before the TVA Travel Board returns to Ft. Harrison."

Vernon's response: "I have the following symptoms with my TMJ. Pain is the most prevalent, unable to open mouth or yawn, clicking or popping on both sides of my jaw, severe headaches, bite that is uncomfortable, neck, shoulder, and back pain, and ringing in my ears. I also suffer from depression due to the pain I suffer from every day. The pain in my jaw is constant; it never lets up. It does not come and go; it is always there. I cannot eat any chewy foods and have to limit my diet to soft or liquid foods...

"I have made arrangements with my employer to work only two hours a day, three to four days a week, at which time I do not take my medication. I cannot work more than two hours because it exceeds my tolerance of the pain and I need to take my medication as soon as I get home. I have to work two hours a day three to four days a week to continue my health coverage for my family, as my wife does not have that benefit option at her employer."

Vernon's last job was with the U.S. Postal Service in Fairfield. "I had terrible headaches and I wasn't very good with customers. Everyone else had all the boxes memorized, but I couldn't remember jack. I could only remember one, and it was my own. That's why I'm unemployed today and living in a trailer in Power [a town north of Great Falls]."

But his job fighting the VA continues. "I still get a letter every month saying they're working on my claims and please be patient. I have three appeals that are waiting to be forwarded to Washington, and they tell me it will be another year and a half before I hear anything on them. I've almost lost my wife and my kids over this, almost taken my own life. If it weren't for all my wife's good work, I'd either have ended it all or be living out in the hills somewhere all by myself."

No longer fit for a job

Many vets have trouble holding down a steady job after their return. Maybe a job just doesn't seem important after all they've been through. Maybe they don't feel they fit in with their co-workers. Maybe they can't focus on work after brutal nights of grueling nightmares and days plagued by flashbacks.

Or maybe it's all of the above.

"I could always get jobs, but I could never hold them. I just couldn't handle the pressure," said Don Scott, a Vietnam vet who had 37 or 38 jobs before he was finally given a 100 percent disability discharge and allowed to retire.

Soon after the 1968 Tet offensive, Scott was sent to Vietnam as an infantryman. "I stopped counting combat experiences at 90," he said. "And that's 90 times in combat, not 90 days. Sometimes you'd get ambushed in the morning and then again in the afternoon, sometimes more than once. I saw a lot of people killed. One of my closest friends sat down on a land mine, and piece of shrapnel went through the back of his head, killing him. I stepped on a land mine — and survived. I don't know how I did it, but I've still got 10 fingers and 10 toes."

He remembers riding a truck and being ordered off it, told to walk instead. "It got ambushed right after that, and six of the seven people on it were killed." That set up a load of survivor guilt, questions of why he survived when his friends didn't, a question that frequently came out in flashbacks.

"I keep on visualizing those guys on the truck that died, my friend dying from sitting on the land mine when I stepped on one and didn't. That made me feel guilty because they died and I didn't."

Sometimes, the dreams are worse. "A lot of them are like the flashbacks, but there are some really gruesome ones that I can't talk about," he said. "I'm watching atrocities and watching them prosecute war crimes. I remember capturing three gooks, putting them on a helicopter that took off. Pretty soon, one of the gooks came out of the chopper. Then another body came out. But the third never fell."

Struggling with those issues, he worked briefly as a carpenter, insurance salesman, janitor, used car salesman, and cleaning supply agent. He also held a number of jobs in heavy construction. "When I was teaching school, the pressure really got to me," he said. "The pain in my leg [nerve damage from shrapnel] was getting worse, and so was the ringing in my ears that I'd been having ever since I stepped on the land mine."

Finally he was given a 100 percent disability, as well as two Purple Hearts for his wounds in Vietnam. "But the one great thing is that my wife has stuck by me for 36 years," he said. He's still in therapy, participating in two group sessions and seeing a counselor and a psychiatrist every week.

Because he has the support of the medical staff, Scott has access to medications to block a lot of his pain. He takes a dozen pills a day. In addition to three ibuprofens for pain and one vitamin B12 for nerve damage, he takes two or three hydrocodones (depending on pain), two or three acetaminophens (depending on pain), one gabapentin, two quetiapine fumarates, one citalopram hydromide, and one trazodone.

- 11 -
Vets in trouble

Faces of Combat who come back damaged by their experiences will continue to haunt us until we find ways to get them integrated back into civilian society. Here is one success and one failure of the system.

Oddly enough, Danny Ray Reed II hit rock bottom at about 20,000 feet in the air, but a federal magistrate's decision to offer help instead of punishment may have saved his life.

A former Army Ranger who'd been involved in the "rescue" of Private 1st Class Jessica Lynch from insurgents in Iraq, Reed was struggling to adjust to civilian life after three years of combat with Special Operations. "When you come back, you're either a workaholic or an alcoholic," he said. "If I wasn't working, I was drinking. It helps for the first couple of hours, but then it takes you back into that frame of mind you don't want to be in. I drank so bad I had two-day blackout, and

149

that's dangerous. Like that airplane incident, I can't remember a thing. I can't remember getting on that plane, and I can't remember getting off. I don't remember that day at all."

That day was Sunday, January 7, 2007, and Reed was flying from his home in West Virginia to Montana, where he had enrolled in a taxidermy school. According to the incident report filed later, when he boarded the United Airlines flight in Denver, "Reed had slurred speech but did not smell of alcohol." It said that an airline attendant served Reed two drinks, but a passenger sitting across the aisle from him, Jolynn Hamilton, a business owner from Lewistown, Montana, observed otherwise. "I believe he purchased from the attendant five bottles of alcohol, Jack Daniels," she wrote to Reed's defense team. "He asked for a cup of ice and asked the flight attendant to pour three bottles of alcohol into his cup of ice, which she did. He immediately 'chugged' down the drink, took the remaining two bottles out of his pocket and asked the attendant to help him open the two bottles and pour them into his glass, which she did. He drank all of it. Within a few minutes, it was obvious that the alcohol took effect — he was very vocal."

According to the incident report, Reed became verbally abusive of other passengers and the attendant began to serve him nonalcoholic drinks. "When Reed figured out that he was not being served alcohol, he threw his drink at [the flight attendant] and told her to 'shove it.'"

It was a tense flight. Police officers were waiting when the plane touched down in Great Falls, and Reed was carted off to jail. He was charged with interfering with aircraft crewmembers, a federal crime that carries a maximum 20-year prison term and $250,000 fine, if convicted. "When I woke up in jail, it was like a nightmare," Reed said. "I didn't know where I was, why I was there, or what I had done. I was scared to death."

From jail, Reed called his folks, Danny Ray, Sr. and Sonja Reed in Lerona, West Virginia, and that turned out to be his saving grace. His mom called the Great Falls *Tribune* and told us all about her son, the war hero, and how he needed treatment instead of punishment. "He never had any trouble before he went into the military, but he came back from the service a different person," she told me. Her calls apparently saved the day. When Reed was arraigned, the chief public defender Tony

Gallagher requested a psychiatric evaluation to look for PTSD and federal magistrate Keith Strong concurred.

That document remains sealed in the federal courthouse, but Reed remembers talking at length about his tours of duty with the Army's 75th Ranger Regiment in Iraq and Afghanistan. Death surrounded him the entire time. "The first thing I saw when I landed in Bagram was a little girl get blown up by a landmine as she was walking her dog," he said. "After that, I saw kids with no arms and no legs. I can't forget the carnage and the smell of war. I've seen people get shot. My friend got half his leg blown off. We got mortared every day."

As a Special Operations unit, the Rangers were given the tough assignments, many of which Reed still can't discuss because they've been classified as top secret. "In Afghanistan, I was in a lot of firefights, doing search and destroy operations," he said. "We were looking for missile launch sites, kidnappers, and [Osama] bin Laden's primary and secondary men." When they needed it, they called in aerial firepower, and Reed still can't get over its shock and awe value. "That AC-130 Spectre is really unreal," he said. "It's unreal how devastating that stuff is and how much damage it can do. I'm speechless how much damage that stuff does." But firepower that awesome can't differentiate between the insurgents and ordinary civilians. "In every war, there are all kinds of kids involved," Reed said.

Reed told the pre-sentencing investigators that he feared the worst when the Rangers were ordered to protect an elite extraction team sent in to rescue PFC Lynch, a member of the 507th Maintenance Company. Lynch had been captured by the insurgents March 23, 2003, as her convoy made a wrong turn into enemy territory and was ambushed near Nasiriyah, a major crossing point over the Euphrates River northwest of Basra. Lynch was injured and captured by Iraqi forces, as were five other soldiers, who were later rescued. Eleven other soldiers were killed in the ambush. Lynch's best friend, Lori Piestewa, was seriously wounded in the head and died in an Iraqi hospital.

The story of the ambush, Lynch's captivity, and her rescue a week later have been so controversial that even Lynch has accused the Department of Defense (and subsequently the news media) of doctoring the truth. Reed, however, remembers that day as much less severe than he had feared. "The briefing for that mission was actually done about 24 hours before it went down, it was that quick. They pounded the objective really hard [with aerial firepower] before we went in. I was with a weapons squad, providing security for all the buildings around the hospital. A group of highly trained soldiers, an elite extraction squad, went in and came out with her in no time at all. We all thought it was going to be a gunfight at the OK Corral, but no bullets were fired."

After Lynch was rescued from the Saddam Hospital in Nasiriyah, however, soldiers had to dig up the bodies of the eight other American soldiers buried behind it. "You could see them and you could smell them," Reed said. "It was awful. It was like the 'Night of the Living Dead.'"

Government agrees that Reed needs help

After Reed recounted what he'd been through, it was obvious the ex-Ranger needed help. "When I took their test, I answered all their questions to the best of my knowledge," he said. "And they said my score was so bad, there was no way I could have that much PTSD."

Prosecutors dropped their request for a prison sentence, and probation officer Kevin Heffernan arranged for treatment at the VA's psychiatric hospital in Fort Sheridan, Wyoming, Judge Strong accepted Reed's guilty plea to a misdemeanor assault charge, put him on probation, and ordered him to report to Fort Sheridan immediately. That turned out to be the best thing they could have done.

"If that plane thing hadn't happened, I'd have probably committed suicide. I'd had a gun in my mouth before. I was at rock bottom. I was so depressed I'd have probably killed myself if that hadn't happened."

Reed remembers Fort Sheridan as an aging Army outpost, underfunded and understaffed. "They're not prepared for the surge of troops that are going to come back needing help," he said. But they sure helped him there. "Step one is admitting that you do have PTSD. And step two was to quit drinking and drugging. They're different in some ways, but PTSD and alcoholism are a lot alike in other ways. You have to admit you have those problems. You can't be in denial about it. And you have to realize that it's something that won't go away, can't be cured. All you can do is learn to live with it."

Reed began to realize he'd brought home a huge load of fear and anger with him. "Things that didn't bother me before I went through the military really bother me now," he said. "People who do stupid things, airheaded things, really bother me because you can't afford to do those things. Being in the military, you're around people a lot and everything seems kind of normal, but when you get home and have time to think, it's very different. I kept on thinking about the things that could have happened, a lot of what ifs? You're by yourself instead of with your military pals. My friends could see a difference in me, but they couldn't understand it, and your good drinking buddies aren't going to take the time to read a pamphlet on PTSD. I felt like people didn't want to be around me. They didn't like me. They're out to get me, talking about me. That went into more drinking, more depression, more seclusion. Then the anger started. I hated these people because they knew nothing about what I'd done, what I'd gone through."

In group therapy, he learned how to talk about his problems and reason them through to a solution. He learned that nightmares and flashbacks are normal and that neither is an excuse to pick up a bottle. And he learned that he has to readjust his thinking to a civilian world.

"Over there, you're in a savage world. It's not civilized. And then when you come back home, this seems out of the ordinary to me. I'm still trying to figure out how to adapt to it," Reed said. "Right now, those savage responses are dormant in me, but I have to realize that they're still there and they can come out if I let them. So I have to walk on a different road. I'd never laid a hand on a girl, but I was drinking and we were arguing and she slapped me. I grabbed her arm, twisted it, and got a chokehold on her. The next day, her arm was all bruised. This girl used to love me, but she told my mom I'm not the same man she knew."

And that baffles Reed, a young man who doesn't feel he has been through anything unusual. "I haven't done half the stuff that a lot of guys have done," he said. "I know guys who are doing their third, fourth, or fifth tours of duty, and they saw way more shit than I did. But the stuff I did see, it sure did do a number on me."

Clean and sober now

When Reed was released from Fort Sheridan, he came back to Montana to study taxidermy. Then he returned to West Virginia, moved in again with his parents, and opened Natural Image, his own taxidermy shop in a building beside the house. Business has been booming for him, with about $15,000 worth of work on order, and he's thinking about expanding. Since he quit drinking, his friends are beginning to hang out with him again.

And Reed is learning to live with a condition that will be with him for the rest of his life. He doesn't like to admit it, but combat has changed the way his brain functions and the doctors have prescribed meds for him that help restore his brain's natural chemistry.

He has been spared flashbacks, but the nightmares still plague him. "Sometimes I dream that all those people who got killed are sitting beside the road, waving at me as we go by," he said. And he told his mom at one point that he dreamed the dead soldiers they unearthed behind the hospital at Nasiriyah were coming back to get him. Reed said, "My dad told me the only two cures for PTSD are Alzheimer's and death, and he should know. He did two tours of 'Nam with the 101st Airborne, and he has PTSD too."

The lesson that we learned from Reed is an important one: treatment can help a vet become productive again. I shudder to think what would have happened if the system had operated normally, without the intervention of Reed's mother. He would probably have been convicted and sent to prison for a couple of years. With a growing sense of rage, he would have gotten into trouble. And when he got out, he would have been a ticking time bomb, a danger to self and to others.

I thought the decision to send Reed off for treatment was a wise one, and it's one that judges around the country should heed. They'll be seeing more and more vets in trouble, and it will be critical to get them help, not jail.

Help must be available to combat vets

In 1981, the federal government conducted a study of 1,000 Vietnam vets who had seen combat. Researchers found that nearly one quarter of them had been arrested since returning home. With the increasing amount of conflict in the past half century and the increasing number of former combat vets in our society, that's a problem that has been increasing.

In January of 2008, the New York *Times* did a nationwide investigation and came up with 121 cases in which combat vets committed a killing, or were charged with one, after returning from war in Iraq or Afghanistan. The *Times* also provided a mug shot of each veteran and a thumbnail account of the murders. That piece of public-service journalism brings the reality of PTSD — described as a combat reaction to a civilian provocation — straight home to the reader.

In America, help is slowly becoming available for combat vets who find difficulty in adjusting to a civilian world. In western Massachusetts, a group called Soldier On has joined other veterans' advocates, mental health experts, and prosecutors to provide training programs for police officers, dispatchers, and other emergency workers. They say it's increasingly common for returned combat veterans to be suicidal, take risks such as extreme speeding, or be involved in domestic disputes. While the group has no statistics on the number of such incidents, it said that's not the point. The point is to try and prevent them.

Most emergency care providers don't know how to differentiate combat vets from other offenders, such as those with mental illnesses. "How you handle a potentially violent situation is going to be the same regardless of the population, since our officers go into it not knowing what's gotten the person worked up," said Audrey Honig, chair of psychological services for the International Association of Chiefs of Police and chief psychologist for the Los Angeles County Sheriff's Department. She told the Associated Press, "It's asking a lot of too few officers to be able to quickly differentiate someone who's an Iraq veteran, or who has bipolar disorder, or who's schizophrenic, or who's just having a really bad day."

The training program gives advice to police officers, firefighters, and others on how to recognize when erratic or defiant behavior results from untreated trauma or brain injuries. In some cases, that can be as simple as defusing a situation so officers can strike up a conversation and determine whether the person is a veteran. Since many police officers are veterans as well, trainers think such conversations can encourage vets to let their guard down and share what's troubling them. In cases where a person is out of control, trainers suggest talking to family members to determine what the problems may be.

Officers are also encouraged to watch for signs of military service such as military-related stickers on cars stopped for traffic violations, wartime pictures in homes where domestic abuses are suspected, or close-cropped hair that hasn't yet begun to grow back.

The experts' advice is to be cautious. Troubled vets should be given ample space, without touching them unless absolutely necessary. Vets may be suffering flashbacks and be confused about where they are and who the officer is. Their attention may be riveted on the officer's weapon. And while they may be acting normally for a combat situation, they don't realize that it's abnormal behavior for a civilian setting.

"It takes a while for these soldiers to stop seeing everything as life-threatening," said Darrell Benson, a veterans' case manager in western Massachusetts. That means that crises must be averted before troubled vets can receive the help they need to deal with their problems.

Prescription painkillers to block the memories

Vets across the country are also watching another case, which also involves a troubled former Army Ranger. He's Sargent Binkley, a decorated former Army captain currently sitting in a San Mateo, California, jail cell on charges that he held up two pharmacies to get the prescription drugs that he'd become addicted to. The former Eagle Scout and West Point graduate is facing a possible prison sentence of no less than 12 years.

Binkley was sent to Bosnia in 1999 where his unit unearthed the mass graves of more than 7,000 Muslim men and boys, the victims of an ethnic genocide campaign four years earlier by Serbs at Srebrenica. It was duty made tougher by the Serbs who clashed with the American forces, hurled bottles and sticks and rocks at them, and bragged loudly about how the evil Muslims got what they deserved.

From Bosnia, Binkley went to the Soto Cano Air Base in Honduras in 2001 to participate in a joint anti-drug campaign. According to a subsequent psychiatric evaluation, he watched one Honduran officer execute three of his own men, apparently believing they were helping the drug runners. On another mission, Binkley said he fired on a Jeep believed to be providing security for a drug operation. Both occupants were killed, but one of them turned out to be a young teenager. Binkley's Web page said, "At one point, he was ordered to open fire on a truck that contained a civilian teenaged boy, an act that haunts him to this day. While on duty in Honduras, he fractured his pelvis and dislocated his hip. The injury was consistently misdiagnosed by Army doctors over the next several years, resulting in chronic pain and an addiction to prescription painkillers."

After his discharge from the Army in 2002, a private sports physician diagnosed the injury and surgery cured it, but he was still left with PTSD and the addiction. In 2006, he concedes that he held up two pharmacies at gunpoint to get the drugs he craved, but he contends that the gun was not loaded. In the first robbery, he gave the pharmacist, Dennis Pinheiro, a list of the painkillers he needed. "He was calm in demeanor and did not use physical or verbal force," Pinheiro wrote in a letter to the court in which he requested leniency for Binkley. "I did as he said and never felt highly threatened, but of course did not want to find out if he could be [violent]." In the second robbery, he told two pharmacy technicians to fill a bag with painkillers, then left with the drugs and these parting words, "Ladies, have a good night."

In California, state law requires a minimum 12-year prison sentence for anyone convicted of using a gun during an armed robbery, and prosecutors don't seem inclined to make an exception. "His life history and the tragedy he's suffered do not outweigh his criminal behavior to the extent that he should be treated any differently than someone else in a similar situation," deputy Santa Clara County district attorney Rob Baker told the San Francisco *Chronicle*. "It ultimately comes down to fairness."

Binkley's Web page is crowded with letters of support. "I have written four letters to the DAs mentioned on this Web page," wrote Judy Boore. "Because I am an embedded counselor in a military unit and have counseled a number of veterans in my private practice, I am aware of the problematic situations they have endured in Iraq, the post-traumatic stress symptoms they bring home and the difficulties they encounter in working with the Veterans Administration. I hope my letters will help the DAs see a bigger picture of a widespread problem [proper care for returning veterans and reintegrating them into the community] and step up to the challenges of finding better solutions for our veterans. I hope the first beneficiary will be Sarge."

This case demonstrates what happens when the system doesn't provide help, and it's heartbreaking to watch. As a nation, we need to recognize that combat damages people and that if we send them abroad to fight for us, we need to take care of them when they come home. Binkley was trying to resolve a medical problem that resulted from his combat experience, and he deserves our help. And it's not just Binkley. It's all around us.

- 12 -

Why are some soldiers more resilient?

Combat vets have different reactions to similar experiences. Researchers are currently working to understand why some vets can bounce back from a traumatic experience that another vet just can't shake. Some of the answers may lie in genetic differences, and some may be a result of earlier childhood trauma.

Memories of Iraq still haunt many members of Montana's 163rd Infantry Battalion. When the battalion left for Iraq in 2004, it was the largest deployment of troops from Montana since World War II. It was also one of the most dangerous combat missions for the Montana Army National Guard unit.

"Every one of my guys except one from the 163rd witnessed IEDs [improvised explosive devices]," said Keli Remus of Chinook Winds

Counseling in Great Falls. "All were shot at or have shot others. All had at least heard of rapes. It seems like every one of my guys was in a vehicle that was blown up, had a friend who was blown up, or had to clean up after a bombing."

Combat exposure checklists consistently show that members of the 163rd experienced moderate to heavy combat in Iraq, said Eric Kettenring, a counselor at the Missoula Vet Center. "And they *are* experiencing trauma, some of it severe, some of it less so, but it's all bad stuff."

America's civilian soldiers also appear to be more vulnerable to combat stress than full-time military personnel.

The Army's leading expert on post-traumatic stress disorder, Col. Charles Hoge, recently told Congress that 41 percent of returning National Guardsmen and Reservists raised concerns about their mental health in a survey taken three to six months after returning from combat. He said one-third of them exhibited symptoms so severe that they were referred for further help. By comparison, one-third of the regular-duty soldiers raised similar concerns, but only 13 percent were referred for further treatment.

"Guard guys have more stress," said Michael Mason, chief counselor at the Center for Mental Health in Great Falls. "Their average age is a little older. They're more established and they're more likely to have families, which creates added stress on the home front."

Members of the 163rd didn't seek any special help in Iraq, nor did they during demobilization at Fort Lewis, Washington. "The 163rd got wind of the fact that some guy in a different unit said yes to some of the debriefing questions and got held back for 30 to 45 days to get counseling," said Remus. "So they all answered no to all the questions because they wanted to get back to see their wives and kids."

And the members of the 163rd are now paying a price for their service (and their denial). "About a third of my guys have a terrible problem with alcohol," Remus said.

But not all, and that's a fascinating issue for researchers. Three soldiers who went through some of the toughest combat say they emerged with problems that appear to be temporary and that they're in the process of shaking off.

Commander's responsibilities

Capt. Mike Beck, former commander of Bravo Company of the 163rd Infantry Battalion in Great Falls, said he knows of six members of his 135-man unit who were diagnosed with PTSD after serving in Iraq for a year. "But I suspect there are more," he added.

Beck recorded in his diary what it felt like to come under fire for the first time.

"As I looked back toward the Humvee just 50 meters in front of us, suddenly there was a huge explosion next to the vehicle," he wrote on December 20, 2004.

"Dirt, fire, smoke, and debris flew a hundred feet in the air as the Humvee disappeared from view. The radio echoed with the chatter of soldiers announcing IED ... IED."

Beck wrote that he was calm during the incident. "It wasn't until everything was over that I noticed my heart was beating rapidly," he wrote.

Six months later, he wrote of the strain of leading his men in a war zone. "It's like having a knot in your stomach every time you leave the wire [compound], thinking this time we'll get hit again. Is it just another dead dog on the side of the road, or does it conceal an artillery round waiting for our approach? Is the next car that approaches us going to swerve into our convoy and explode, or will it be like the hundreds of others that just roll by? As we travel, how many eyes staring at me wish I were dead? As I walk through a village, does a sniper have his scope trained on my head? Is it trained on the head of one of my soldiers? Did the explosion I just heard in the distance injure a soldier?

"What is it like here? It sucks. I'm ready for my soldiers to go home," he wrote on May 20, 2005.

Beck said a combat stress team routinely offered assistance to his soldiers every two or three months while they were in Iraq. "And they made a pretty good effort to show up every time there was significant activity," he added. There was a mental stress exam when soldiers demobilized in Fort Lewis, he said, although he knew of no one singled out for help.

"There were a lot of close calls," Beck said. "We saw a lot of things that were disturbing, not only the dead and wounded allies, but also the dead and wounded Iraqis, especially if you were responsible for their condition."

Beck seemed to adjust well, but a couple of months after his return, he began having vulnerability nightmares in which he was leaving his base camp in Iraq in a Humvee without armor, without a weapon, or without his own body armor. "I'd awake a little disturbed until I realized I was home," he said.

Bombing victim

"Almost all of us come back with issues," said Staff Sgt. Adam Bell, who works for the National Guard in Helena. "Half of us do get help for issues large and small, a quarter of us fight it, and a smaller percentage just don't know what do to about it."

Bell, a gunner aboard an armored Humvee, completed more than 100 combat missions, was bombed 10 times, and came under fire a couple of times. "On August 19, 2005, I was hit by an IED near Hawijah," he said. "It struck the right side of the vehicle, and I took shrapnel to my left leg and right foot."

Ten surgeries and a bone graft later, he walks without a noticeable limp.

"When I was released from the hospital, I don't think I slept for the first month," Bell said. "I think it was due to the quietness. You're surrounded by noise in Iraq."

Nightmares were a problem, but they're finally diminishing. "I dreamed I was back in the truck going through that explosion again," said Bell. "I could smell everything, hear everything, touch everything, and taste everything. It's pretty weird."

Bell said he has received excellent medical care and psychiatric counseling from the Veterans Administration. "A soldier has to recognize that there's something wrong and have the courage to ask for help," he said. "Just like my foot, my brain can be fixed. And that means I can continue my military career."

Unexpected deployment

"I think a lot of guardsmen never thought they'd go into combat," said Staff Sgt. Tim Colvin of Butte, Montana. Colvin had an uncle who retired from the National Guard after 25 years of easy stateside duty, so he figured it was a good way to get through college. "But after two deployments, I realize the times are changing," he said.

Colvin served first in Bosnia. In Iraq, Colvin's Humvee was bombed 13 times. The 13th was definitely unlucky. "We were hit by two 152mm howitzer rounds that blew up, kind of like a bombshell," he said. "It shredded my Humvee, blew off my back driver's side door, ripped my door open, and threw some shrapnel inside."

Colvin was left with head injuries and a leg so badly shredded that shrapnel broke the bone. As the doctors in Fort Lewis worked to put Colvin back together, so did the psychiatrists. "I had problems with not knowing what happened to my guys," he said. "I had a feeling that I'd let them down by not getting them home safely."

Nightmares of explosions kept him awake. They persisted until April or May. "I didn't sleep at all," said Colvin. "I had some sleeping pills, but they never helped."

Flashbacks came at unexpected times. He's still troubled by the terrorists who would strap a family in a car as decoys, then blow up the car as a convoy passed by. "There was a little six-year-old kid in a car who was severely injured," Colvin said. "It was particularly hard because I had a kid that age. The fact that they would do something like that was just mind-boggling."

His symptoms have diminished a bit since he married again a couple of years ago, Colvin said, but his new wife still has to wake him up when he gets to yelling and swearing and thrashing in the middle of the night. "I don't think there are enough counselors out there who really understand the effects of war and what soldiers are coming back with," he said. "It took a long time for my counselors to understand what I'd been through."

Studying resilience in soldiers

But the ability to go through combat experiences like these and shake off the emotional disorders that paralyze some soldiers fascinates — and perplexes — researchers. Many suspect the answer is a combination of environmental and genetic factors that seem to co-exist in the mind. For example, some people are predisposed genetically to become alcoholics, but environmental stressors push them over that edge.

Such mental illnesses seem to be like the Gateway Arch in St. Louis. An arch stands over each one of us — no one is immune. One leg of the arch is *genetic*. As others in your family suffer from alcoholism or mental illness, you can pretty well chart the increasing risk to yourself. And the other leg is *environmental*. As you face increasing environmental stressors, things like job insecurity or failing relationships or the cruel certainty that even your dog no longer loves you, you may be tempted to self-medicate with alcohol or drugs, or to hide away in mental fantasies/delusions. And combat can be a major stressor.

So why are some soldiers able to rise above these threats? Researchers have long believed that some people are more *resilient*, a term meaning that they are capable of implementing early, efficient adjustment processes to alleviate strain imposed by exposure to stress, thus allowing to body to return to its normal balance after a temporary disturbance.

Some environmental factors can aid resilience. Since trauma builds on itself, those unscarred by childhood trauma will be stronger under combat. Social support is important, and those who have a community of family or friends will be more likely to survive. Attitude is important; those who believe they can handle the worst will stand a better chance of doing so, and those who don't feel hopeless will always benefit from their can-do attitude.

Biological factors can be equally positive. One of those factors is the way you process emotions. Some people panic and go to pieces, while others master their fear and funnel it into preventive and protective action. One genetic difference is the serotonin transporter gene, the mechanism that sucks excess serotonin from the synapse (gap) after it passes an electrical impulse from one synaptic nerve to the next. Some people have a pair of larger, more efficient serotonin transporter genes that recapture more of the neurotransmitter. Since serotonin has been closely related to mood swings and anxiety attacks, as well as regulation of sleep and aggression, better control in your brain cells may mean better control of your emotions. People with the long genes are more resilient, while those with the short genes are more likely to experience depression and suicidal behavior. While that's been proven in mental illness, researchers have recently found that it also carries over to PTSD.

Another difference is a gene that produces an amino acid neurotransmitter called neuropeptide-Y (NPY). Vets with combat-related PTSD have been found to have lower baseline levels of NPY, and their NPY doesn't work as effectively in controlling stress. Studies of military personnel exposed to extreme stress have found that higher levels of NPY seem to block some of the symptoms of dissociation, an emotional numbing and a likely source for dissociative flashbacks among vets. By calming the amygdala, the emotional "fight-or-flight" center, NPY also appears to improve the ability of the cortex to reason — or perhaps it just strengthens the cortex in reining in the amygdala. So far, no medication has been developed that can enhance this natural process.

Researchers are looking at another neurotransmitter known as DHEA, which is found in the adrenal cortex. There's a body of evidence that trauma causes production of the stress hormone cortical, which sends a red-flag warning to the rest of the brain. It seems to promote increased arousal, vigilance, focused attention, and emotional memory formation. It also mobilizes and replenishes high-energy supplies. All of these are designed to be only a temporary response to a threat — prolonged overstimulation can lead to cell damage or death. "DHEA seems to reduce the stress that the cortical is associated with," Dr. Matthew Friedman, director of the VA's National Center for PTSD, told me. "The ability to mobilize DHEA is another way to increase resilience. The question is whether NPY and DHEA are fellow travelers, or whether people are able to mobilize one or the other."

New research in Atlanta

A new study out of Emory University in Atlanta suggests that some people may be at higher genetic risk of PTSD. In fact, one gene alone may make them twice as vulnerable.

A team of researchers led by Dr. Kerry Ressler examined 900 adults, mostly middle-aged, low-income African-Americans who had suffered both childhood and adult abuse. The team looked at a stress gene called FKBP5, which regulates a portion of the adrenal gland. It's the adrenal gland that produces cortisol and adrenaline. Both are involved in the flight-or-fight syndrome, created when the brain's hypothalamus senses a threat that a human being must react to. The FKBP5 gene produces a protein (not a hormone) called a "chaperone" that helps the cortisol receptor function. When it's involved with the inhibitory process rather than the excitatory, it's responsible for shutting down the cortisol after the threat has been averted.

Ressler's team found that there are at least two variants of this particular gene, although there may be more, he said. Scientists aren't yet able to tell how the genes differ because research is still in the early stages. "This is currently at the level of 'we now know that this gene is involved in an interesting way,' but the details for how it is involved are not yet clear," Ressler told me. "It will probably take years of basic research to figure it out fully."

One thing is now clear: the genetic variants do an uneven job in returning the neurosystem to normal. Some people who suffered the same sorts of trauma ended up with twice the symptoms of PTSD, said Ressler. "The end result of such findings would be that it might be possible to determine in advance who would be most vulnerable to PTSD. The 'effect size' of this gene is probably not large enough in itself to ever be predictive by itself, but in the future combined with other risk and resilience genes and with measures of psychological variables that also mediate risk, one could potentially determine some level of risk pre-trauma. With that, and a further understanding of the biology, these data may one day help block PTSD formation following a trauma in those at risk."

What Dr. Ressler is saying is that while one gene can be proven to make a difference, it's not acting alone. It's acting in conjunction with many other genes in a very complex interaction, which we cannot yet begin to understand. And that reminds me of what Dr. Javier Castellanos, one of the leading researchers into attention deficit hyperactivity disorder (ADHD), told me when I visited him at the National Institute of Mental Health in Bethesda, Maryland, several years ago. He said he had been able to find no single genetic cause of ADHD and had begun to fear that it was a subtle malformation of a number of genes, which could explain the wide range of symptoms. If that's the case, Castellanos said, it could take decades of research to understand and treat ADHD. I suspect the same will be true of PTSD.

- 13 -
State of denial

Ask a soldier if he or she has a problem and the soldier will almost always say, "No, I can handle it." The Faces of Combat look in a mirror and have trouble seeing what has happened to them. To help our veterans we need to get past their denial and the denial of our health care system.

Denial is a huge part of the problem. Members of the National Guard or Reserves don't want to talk about their problems.

Some of it is a cultural thing. Soldiers are supposed to be tough, able to get through just about anything. They don't want to admit their fear, so they repress it. They also bond with members of their unit — their lives are in each other's hands — and they don't want to do anything that would damage that relationship. In particular, they don't want to step away when a buddy may need them.

Frequently, there's a second underlying motive for this denial. The National Guard or the Reserves is a paying second job, and many families have come to rely on that income. Sometimes, vets have lost their primary job — or a spouse who brought in a second paycheck — and that money becomes more critical.

Active-duty soldiers believe their careers will be jeopardized if they become diagnosed with PTSD. And there are just enough horror stories floating around to justify those fears.

One of those horror stories is that of Sgt. David Lee Davies.

Davies was active-duty with the U.S. Navy from 1988-90 and saw action in the conflict with Libya, shooting down several of its jets. He now lives in Illinois, but has been a member of the Iowa National Guard since 1995. In 2003, his unit was deployed to Iraq and was in combat for 15 months due to an involuntary extension of its tour of duty under a presidential stop-loss order.

He told me that his first job was at a forward observation post, FOB Iceberg, where his job was to get information on the insurgents from local residents. "We'd go out from the base camp, wander around, meet them, and win over their hearts and minds. Over time, they would invite us for dinner or tea," said Davies. "We'd help them get their troubles taken care of. We developed really good relationships with the locals. We helped with irrigation. We never had a problem. The locals took very good care of us. The problem is third-country nationals."

Over time, that relationship soured. "About four months after the President announced we were done fighting offensive operations, the problems started. They saw us sitting back on our heels. We had become a static army, which was not a good thing to be. The locals started asking us when we were going to leave, and when we said we didn't know, then they began to get angry."

After that, Davies began escorting convoys, which were prime targets for insurgents. "I don't remember my personal actions in combat," he said. "I've blocked them out. I know I fired my weapon because I had to clean it. I know I ran out of ammunition. My wife was on the phone with me when we got into a firefight, so I know it happened. And my driver Yonie told me when we got into a firefight, I'd be yelling 'Get some.'"

His wife Terry remembers those firefights well. "There were many times when I was on the phone with David and he forgot to hang up with me or just went into that mode," she said. "I heard him shooting and then I could hear more shots, and then a few minutes later, he got back on the phone and started talking to me like nothing happened."

When Davies returned from Iraq, Terry knew immediately there was something wrong. "As soon as he came back, it wasn't diagnosed, but I was aware of the impulsive behavior in thinking and actions like shopping, instant gratification. He was very controlled."

In February 2006, the couple went to Fort Benning, Georgia, to find out what was wrong with him. "The first appointment didn't find that much wrong, but the second was for chronic PTSD," Terry said. "They said he would never be able to work again. I turned to the doctor in total shock and said, 'Are you trying to tell me there's no help for him?' and the doctor told me, 'That's exactly what I'm telling you.'"

Davies is still trying to get back to normal, but finding that middle ground elusive. "My psychiatrists tell me I'm repressing all those memories, and that's where my problems are coming from. They've thrown medication at me. I don't have any mood swings any more, but some of the medications just make me feel like a zombie."

As soon as he notified his National Guard unit of his disability, he said his status there changed immediately. "I became a janitor because I can't carry a weapon or put a helmet on or doing any training," said Davies. "My career is over and now I'm just a nuisance that has to be dealt with. Ultimately, I understand. I'm used up. I don't want anyone else to have to go over there and get these memories and have to live with themselves."

That broke Terry's heart. "They made him clean and shine the armory floors," she said. "He is a man with over 13 years experience and has been to war twice and they have reduced him to that. He has been told that because of his PTSD, he cannot carry a weapon so the unit doesn't know what to do with him."

Struggling with those issues only made things worse. "We've been pushing for counseling, but it didn't happen," Terry said. "A week or so ago, we went to the psychiatric clinic and demanded we get help. We sat there for four hours, and he finally raised his voice. That was his way of exploding. We finally got to see someone, but that's about all we've been able to do."

Although Davies has become resigned to the loss of his military career, his wife feels strongly that he's been wronged. She wants to straighten the whole mess out, but doesn't know how. "This is not the way our soldiers should get treated for all they did when they finish their usefulness because they are sick now from their tours of duty," she said.

Struggling to stay on

Another soldier trying to tough his way through the pain is Sgt. 1st Class Drew Brown, a drill sergeant for the Pennsylvania National Guard. "I'm one of the guys wearing a big stupid hat who walks around and teaches kids how to be soldiers," he said.

Figuring his skills would be useful in Iraq, Brown volunteered to go overseas to help train the Iraqi Army. That turned out to be an assignment that was, to put it mildly, challenging. "Their sense of responsibility and work ethic were wildly different from ours, so if you looked at it through American eyes, you'd be tremendously disappointed," he said. "If you looked at it through Iraqi eyes, however, they were moderately OK. For the first few months, most of my conversations began with 'Hey, asshole.' Later I came to the realization that they were merely doing things in their own way, which could sometimes be more effective than the American way, so my conversations would begin with, 'Hey, buddy' or 'Hey, man.'"

Brown was working with an Iraqi battalion of about 700 soldiers and officers, first trying to recapture the town of Fallujah and later to provide security. Later, his unit was transferred to Taji, a tiny town with a huge military base that had a tank-retrofitting center. "There were a lot of things on the base to go boom," said Brown. "I petitioned the American commander to allow us to begin securing the region around the base. We needed greater security, but I also needed the Iraqi officers and soldiers to be doing something. With 700 soldiers, there are only so many you can keep busy without their getting bored and doing stupid things."

Brown is fairly sure that his tactic reduced the American death toll. His team entered a small village south of the base that appeared friendly during the day, but was suspected of being an insurgent staging area at night. "We conducted a number of house-to-house and field-to-farm searches for munitions," he said. "One particular search found 76 mortar rounds, about 45 107mm rockets, some heavy machine guns, as well as electrical devices that could very easily have been used as triggering devices."

In Baqubah, his unit was charged with blocking roads at random, then doing vehicle-to-vehicle searches. "Things that would terrify most Americans were normal daily occurrences for me," Brown said. "The threat of indirect fire was nerve-racking at first, but I quickly realized they couldn't hit the broad side of a barn if they tried. The most overpowering emotions were anger when they shot at us and frustration when you couldn't bring our forces to bear against them. So frustration and anger were dominant. Fear was there, too, but you can't let fear control you. You acknowledge it, but put it in your pocket to deal with it later."

Asking for help

When Brown returned home from Iraq, he decided he'd do things differently than when he returned home from Bosnia. "Then I tried to find my way home in a bottle. There were few vet services, and the VA was notoriously difficult to deal with." So this time, he asked for help up front in the post-deployment forms he filled out when he left the Iraqi combat theatre, as well as the forms within 30, 90, and 180 days of his return. "I filled out those forms five or six times," he said. "One of the last questions is whether you want to see a mental health professional. I prudently said I did because I thought I might deal with it better now that I was older. But they never contacted me. I had a sense of frustration with society, and I was in a low state — I'd had the barrel of my pistol in my mouth twice. So I called the civilian head of my health program and said I'd never seen a mental health professional. He told me he'd closed my case out. I told him that he'd failed me, that I had had the barrel of my pistol in my mouth and I had to have my case reopened."

That got the VA's attention, and he began to receive help. But most of it, he found, was not very helpful. "One psychologist wanted me to meditate, but I decided meditation sounded like prayer, so I'd stick with that. Another gave me pills to remove my anxiety but neglected to mention that one of the side effects could be depression. After a week of taking the pills, I decided again that there was no reason to go on living. Luckily, I realized that was the drug talking, so I quit taking the pills. The last time I saw the doc, all he wanted to talk about was his vacation in Peru, nothing that impacted me in any way."

So now, he's trying to deal with survivor guilt on his own. "Any number of us vets are dealing with the sense of guilt that you survived, but others didn't," he said. "A fellow drill sergeant who was absolutely a great human being and a friend was killed in December of 2004, and I still miss him to this day. Certain days, I feel this incredible sense of guilt — why Paul and not me? All I can do is chalk it up to the Lord's will, that He has a mission for me and I have to figure out what it is."

Unlike many vets, Brown actually finds some relief in his work because he figures he may be able to teach some of the recruits how to survive in combat. "And the biggest thing I've found is working with other vets through the IAVA [Iraq and Afghanistan Veterans of America] because we've been able to champion some causes. And that's been a big help to me in dealing with my stress. I had a pretty significant flashback that woke me up out of my sleep a week ago, but for the most part, I've learned what kinds of things trigger the flashbacks and I either avoid them or I hit them head on. But I'm not taking meds anymore. I have little confidence that the VA will be able to prescribe me anything that will help me."

Over the past few years, I've talked with a lot of soldiers and counselors who have told me privately that denial is a huge problem for our soldiers. With few exceptions, no one wants to talk about it on the record. They fear that admitting a problem will cost them their job or their friendships, and they aren't willing to take that risk. So they suffer in silence. But there's a big danger in bottling up mental health problems. Untreated, they get worse. And they'll worsen dramatically with further trauma.

Mercifully, the stigma is lessening a little, and soldiers are more willing today to discuss PTSD than they had been just five years ago. But it remains a huge problem, and the military culture only makes it worse.

- 14 -
Disposable veterans

To a combat vet already in physical and emotional pain, it often appears that they have to fight unsympathetic bureaucracies purposely denying them benefits for injuries received in service to their country. Sometimes that's just a perception, but all too often that's true. And if it's only one time, that's still too often.

The Veteran's Disability Benefits Commission, a 13-member congressional commission, spent two and a half years studying disability payments and concluded its 554-page report in the fall of 2007 by saying the government falls woefully short in providing adequate mental health care, as well as timely and fair disability payments.

"Congress should increase the compensation rates up to 25 percent as an interim and baseline future benefit for loss of quality of life, pending development and implementation of quality of life measures," the report stated. "In particular, the measure should take into account the quality of life and other non-work related effects of severe disabilities on veterans and family members."

The commission reported that America had 23.5 million veterans living in the United States and Puerto Rico in 2007, which is about eight percent of the nation's population. With the World War II vets dying off, those numbers have been decreasing for about a decade. Between 2000 and 2004, the size of our veteran population shrank by an average of 437,000 people a year, or 1,200 vets a day. By the end of 2006, Vietnam vets were the largest group in the veteran population. The average age of veterans today is 58 years old, and the majority are between 45 and 64.

But the effects of the current war are beginning to show. More than 2.7 million vets had service-related disabilities at the end of fiscal year 2006, a 14 percent increase from fiscal 2002. And the VA is not geared up to handle that, so vets needing help get punishment instead.

Emotional disabilities can show up as behavioral problems, and vets say the Army tends to discipline the behavior rather than help with the disability. "Some of them have come back and found the capability of accessing services is not immediately available and they've adopted coping mechanisms," said Steve Robinson, a disabled Special Forces vet who heads Veterans for America in Washington, DC. "That translates into a discipline problem for the DOD, so they get kicked out. Their drug abuse and substance abuse programs are all one-strike programs — if you screw up, you're out. So a lot of these guys will end up behind bars."

Discipline can be doubly counter-productive because soldiers thrown out of the Armed Forces with less-than-honorable discharges lose military benefits, including access to VA health care. From 2000 through 2006, the commission found that 69.2 percent of the soldiers received honorable discharges, while 5.6 percent received general discharges under honorable conditions and 6.7 percent received bad conduct or less-than-honorable discharges. Oddly, 18.5 percent of the discharges could not be characterized or were unknown. Basically, that's a way of denying help to the very people who need it the most, a terrible thing to do to our soldiers.

Robinson is also unhappy with the government's response to the mental health needs of its veterans. "There are a lot of people who are trying to get out of paying the cost of mental health care in this country," he said.

One way of doing that is to determine that a vet came into military service with a pre-existing mental disorder. That gets the government off the hook for some of the disability ratings. Since 2001, 22,500 soldiers have been discharged from military service with what's diagnosed as a personality disorder. The Department of Defense Task Force on Mental Health found that personality disorder discharges have increased 40 percent in the Army since the invasion of Iraq, and there's some concern that soldiers suffering from PTSD or TBI may have been pressured by commanders and doctors to accept an administrative discharge rather than stand up for their rights. U.S. Rep. Bob Filner, chairman of the House VA Committee, said, "My concern is that this country is regressing and again ignoring the legitimate claims of PTSD in favor of the time- and money-saving diagnosis of personality disorder."

That's another cop-out that I ran into several times interviewing soldiers for this book. Several of them told me they were discharged with a diagnosis of a personality disorder they never knew they had. By the time they got that news, they were generally so tired that they didn't fight it. And they shouldn't have to. The VA ought to appoint an ombudsman to go back and double check every diagnosis of personality disorder coming out of this war to make sure there's a valid reason for believing that the Army accepted the soldier in that condition.

Despite the undercutting diagnoses, Robinson noted the prevalence of PTSD is spiraling. The Department of Defense had originally estimated that 17 percent of its soldiers would suffer emotional disorders, but upgraded that figure to 35 percent and later to 40 percent. "It's on a plane of going upward, perhaps to 50 or 60 percent," he said.

The commission hoisted a red flag for PTSD, noting that the number and cost of PTSD cases is increasing faster than any other disability. From fiscal 1999 to 2004, it said, "While the total number of all veterans receiving disability compensation grew by only 12.3 percent, the number of PTSD cases grew by 79.5 percent, increasing from 120,265 cases in FY 1999 to 215,871 cases in FY 2004. During the same period, PTSD benefits increased 148.8 percent from $1.72 billion to $4.28 billion. While veterans being compensated for PTSD represented only 8.7

percent of all claims, they received 20.5 percent of all compensation benefits."

The commission said that as of September 2005, the number of vets with PTSD on VA disability rolls had risen to 244,846, requiring monthly payments of $34,867,708. Treatment had been provided to 346,000 veterans overall, meaning that more than 70 percent of them remained disabled as of September 2005. "This means that PTSD is by far the costliest disability for the VA Disability Compensation Program," it concluded. PTSD is marked by high rates of co-morbidity, the commission noted, making assessment difficult. Substance abuse is frequently found with PTSD, as are major depression and anxiety disorders.

Robinson has mixed feelings about the way the Department of Defense handles the medical needs of returning soldiers. "DOD really deals with anger management by medicating them," he said. That's a complaint I've heard from a number of vets, who say the system deals with their problems by throwing pills at them.

Robinson also argues that the VA tries to separate substance abuse from PTSD therapies, requiring that soldiers be substance free before they can begin treating stress disorders. "Last night at 2:30, I got a call from a mother in Georgia telling me that her son is trying to get into the VA for help with his PTSD, but they won't let him in the doors because of substance abuse problems. They said he has to get substance abuse treatment first, and this mother is afraid her son is going to die."

The commission recommended that an overall assessment system be created to provide help uniformly for our vets. And it strongly recommended better data keeping on the condition of vets coming forward with claims, as well as tracking them better after a disability decision had been reached. "There are no easy solutions," it concluded. "Experience with civilian benefits has shown that the problem will be difficult to remedy."

Vet feels the system abused him

VA takes a lot of heat — much of it justified, but not all of it — for the way it treats veterans. It's filled with well-meaning people, but it's also vastly underfunded and clogged with red tape. In that respect, it's a reflection of the Armed Forces it was designed to serve.

Stacey Hayward told me that the military/VA system took advantage of him. It used him while he was fit, but when he got injured, it pushed him aside. "They treated me very poorly," Hayward said. "They wouldn't do anything to help me, gave me every bullshit detail they could and used all kinds of excuses to keep me from getting help."

On September 12, 2001, the day after the terrorist attacks, Hayward left high school, walked into the recruiter's office and signed on the line. "I was ticked that the terrorists attacked us, wanted to defend my country, and decided that was the day to do it," said the 23-year-old Butte native. Hayward ended up in Iraq with the 82nd Airborne Division, where he said he was regularly mortared, bombed, and shot at. "We had all kinds of IEDs [improvised explosive devices], and I lost a couple of friends to them," he said. "And we had a few convoys blown up and had to rescue people or put out fires or remove important equipment. A lot of snipers shot at me, but none of them hit me."

One night while he was on guard duty and taking incoming fire, one member of his squad was shot in the leg and four others severely burned when a sniper's bullet ignited a gas tank. "Our squad leader got burned the worst," said Hayward. "He was brought in while I was there, but I didn't know it was him. I could just see the blood dripping off the truck when they brought him in. I didn't know it was my squad, but I found out the next morning. I was lying in bed and they put the bloody boots of the guy who'd been shot in the leg on the cot next to mine."

That's the stuff of which post-traumatic stress disorder is made, and Hayward told me he began reliving those traumas through flashbacks and nightmares. "The mortars are a big part of my PTSD, too," he said. "I almost got hit by a couple of rockets and a couple of mortars."

When his unit got back stateside, Hayward knew he needed help. "They asked us to fill out a [mental health] questionnaire, and I said I needed help with nightmares and flashbacks," he said. "A couple of my friends said they were feeling suicidal. We turned in our questionnaires, and no one even asked us about it, so we got no help."

Instead, the unit was told it needed to catch up on the parachute jumps it had missed while in combat in Iraq. "I got injured on the second jump through a thunder-and-lightning storm with winds higher than we should have been jumping in and altitudes lower than we should have been jumping in," he said. "I was unconscious for a long period of time. When I rejoined my unit, they told me to tough it out. Then the next morning, they tried to put me on a detail to prevent me from going to the medics."

He did see a medic, however, who diagnosed whiplash and lower back pain. The doc prescribed three days in a darkened room for the concussion, Hayward said. "But they called me into work every single one of those days."

After seven months of working in pain, he said, he was accused of malingering. To prove there was nothing wrong with him, they ordered an X-ray that revealed a P-12 burst fracture — "That's pretty much where the vertebrae explodes under compression," said Hayward — plus a couple of compressed disks. "I finally got out with a medical discharge in January 2006," he said, "but it took close to a year before the VA could work me into its treatment program."

Before his discharge, he said, his medical history vanished from his Army records and he had to go back and prove that he had served overseas and received commendations. And he had to fight to prove that his broken back was the result of the parachute jump, not an auto accident that occurred later when another driver turned into his vehicle at less than 40 mph.

"During that time, I was in a car wreck and the Army tried to blame my broken back on the auto wreck instead of on the jump," he said. "The paperwork continued to be screwed up, including my exit paperwork, so I don't have any of my awards and commendations. It just said I was in the military from this date to that date. And since I couldn't prove I'd been in Iraq, it made it harder to get my PTSD covered by VA."

Some of that has been taken care of, but not all. He's tried to go back to school, but found that the pain of sitting in a classroom sent him to bed for days at a time. And he said he was denied back surgery on the grounds that he wasn't a good candidate for it.

"I'm currently unemployed, have no income except for my disability pay, which is $570 a month, and I think I'm looking at about $5,700 in debt," Hayward said.

Now he's back living with his family in Butte. "It's irritating to me because I'm not used to begging for help," he said. "But I don't have any other choice."

The lawyers move in

There have been so many cases like Hayward's that something had to be done. Hard on the heels of the commission's report came a lawsuit against the VA filed by two veterans' organizations: Veterans for Common Sense in Washington, DC, and Veterans United for Truth in Santa Barbara, California.

"This lawsuit stems from the shameful failure of the United States Department of Veterans Affairs and other governmental institutions to meet our nation's legal and moral obligations to honor and care for our wounded veterans who have served our country," it said. "Because of those failures, hundreds of thousands of men and women who have suffered grievous injuries fighting in the ongoing wars in Iraq and Afghanistan are being abandoned. Unless systematic and drastic measures are instituted immediately, the cost to these veterans, their families, and our nation will be incalculable, including broken families, a new generation of unemployed and homeless veterans, increases in drug abuse and alcoholism, and crushing burdens on the health care delivery system and other social services in our community.

"The system for deciding VA claims has largely collapsed. The VA claims adjudication system is currently mired in processing a backlog of over 600,000 claims, many of which have been pending for years. The time period for a claim to be fully decided can exceed 10 years. By comparison, the private sector health care industry processes 30 billion claims annually in an average of 89.5 days per claim, including the time required to resolve disputed claims. The VA's process for pursuing a claim is not merely arbitrary and ineffective. The delays have become an insurmountable barrier, preventing many veterans from obtaining health care and benefits. Many wounded veterans, particularly those with combat-caused mental illness, give up in frustration and despair or die while their claims are pending. In these cases, justice delayed is justice denied."

PTSD has become a particular challenge for the VA, said the lawsuit. "Veterans with PTSD are among the troops who have suffered the worst due to the disintegration of the VA's claims system. The Iraq and Afghanistan wars have produced an unprecedented number of veterans suffering from this mental disorder. PTSD is prevalent among troops returning from the current wars because of multiple rotations into combat, the absence of battle lines, widespread use of improvised explosive devices, the moral ambiguity of killing combatants dressed as civilians, the unprecedented use of National Guard and Reserve troops, and the use of body armor that saves lives, but leaves minds and bodies shattered...."

PTSD is a cumulative disorder. It worsens with increased exposure to combat. And the wars in Iraq and Afghanistan have provided the greatest cumulative exposure ever, according to the lawsuit.

"In the OEF/OIF, troops are serving longer and more frequent tours of duty than in past conflicts. Many troops have been deployed three or four times and have had their tours of duty involuntarily extended. A considerable number of troops are conducting combat operations every day of the week, 10 to 12 hours per day, for months on end. At no time in military history have large numbers of troops been required to serve on the front line of any war for a period of six or seven months, let alone a year or more, without a significant break to recover from the physical, psychological, and emotional demands that ensue from combat. During WWII, entire units were withdrawn from the line for months at a time in order to rest and recuperate. Even during Vietnam, week-long combat patrols in the field were typically followed by several days of rest and recuperation at the base camp."

Like the claims processing system, the VA's health care system has also collapsed with the drastic increase in demand for services, particularly in the area of mental health, leaving the promise of treatment for wounded soldiers a hollow one, according to the lawsuit. "Veterans tell horror stories not only of having to wait weeks and sometimes months for PTSD treatment, but of insufficient and overworked staff and the absence of any mental health care treatment in rural areas. Although returning troops are statutorily entitled to two years of free care, many never receive any care before the two years elapse."

The lawsuit noted that of the 1,400 VA hospitals and clinics, only 27 offered inpatient treatment for PTSD.

"Perhaps most shamefully, federal government officials have induced many service members suffering from service-related PTSD to accept 'personality disorder' discharges which preclude affected veterans from obtaining disability benefits or receiving ongoing medical treatment because they are classified as having a 'pre-existing condition.' More than 22,500 soldiers across the armed forces have been suspiciously diagnosed and discharged with 'personality disorders' in the last six years, condemning them to a lifetime of disability without compensation or access to VA medical care," it continued.

According to the lawsuit, the number of "personality disorder discharges" increased from 805 in 2001 to 980 in 2003 and nearly 1,100 in 2006. Such "Chapter 5-13" discharges save the government money. "By discharging troops under Chapter 5-13, as opposed to diagnosing them with PTSD, the military will likely save upward of $8 billion in estimated disability payments and $4.5 billion in medical care over the course of the service members' lifetimes."

The lawsuit charged that the VA ties incentive payments to a system of credits for work performed, rewarding adjudicators who process claims more quickly. "As the VA has known for many years, the VA's compensation system has allowed its employees to commit fraud and 'game' the system. VA employees have developed and perfected a number of administrative schemes designed to exploit the system of incentive compensation and artificially enhance their productivity statistics. One of the most common abuses is to prematurely issue a denial decision before the required factual development of a claim is initiated or completed; a second work credit can be garnered if the claim is reopened by the veteran or if an appeal results in a remand for further development. Other abuses include the removal of medical examination reports from claim files, physical alteration of claim files, doctoring of transcripts, and a wide assortment of improper actions...."

The destruction, alteration, and forgery of veterans' records and claim files and other illegal practices continue to this day. The 2006 VA IG Report lists comments from VA staff such as: "For the past 10 years, no examination has been allowed to be returned as inadequate because the regional office concocted a deal with the hospital to cook the books on examination quality.... Rating specialists and DROs [Decision Review Officers] have been pressured to make rating decisions unwarranted by the evidence to make 'problem cases' go away."

The lawsuit concluded that the federal government has callously denied the VA sufficient funding to meet its promises. "The VA's failure to satisfy its statutory mandates to provide health care and disability benefits to disabled veterans has been exacerbated by a deliberate and chronic pattern of underfunding. While the government continues to pay lip service to assisting wounded veterans, the VA has been chronically understaffed and left without the resources or procedures necessary to fulfill the nation's commitment to veterans. The abandonment by the VA of Iraq and Afghanistan veterans and the failure to promptly and properly treat them is penny-wise and pound-foolish. If unredressed, these illegal actions and practices will create another generation of indigent and homeless men and women with staggering social costs."

Early in 2008, a federal judge in San Francisco cleared the way for the lawsuit to proceed as a national class-action challenge to the VA's treatment of soldiers with PTSD. The federal system for weighing individual veterans' claims "does not provide an adequate alternative remedy for plaintiffs' claims," concluded U.S. District Judge Samuel Conti in a 42-page ruling.

After the decision was released, the vets' lead attorney Melissa Kasnitz said: "VA first mistreated hundreds of thousands of veterans, then took the position that the vets could not bring their grievances to court to be heard. Today, VA's shameful effort to keep these deserving veterans from their day in court was rejected."

Personally, I've never been a fan of lawsuits, preferring to negotiate a fair settlement in good faith wherever possible. But the VA is too big, too bureaucratic, and too indifferent for any individual to deal with, to say nothing of a soldier in pain battling crippling emotional disorders. So in this case, I'm delighted to see someone standing up for the vets and using the power of our legal system to force accountability. We're lucky to have a legal system that we can turn to when all else fails. And beyond that, there's the power of the press to mobilize public opinion. Just look at the firestorm that erupted after news reports of the shoddy and dangerous conditions at the Walter Reed Medical Center in Washington, DC.

Under public scrutiny

One national magazine, *The Nation*, has done a commendable job in bringing these outrages to public attention. Last year, it featured the story of Spec. Jon Town, who was wounded in Iraq, received a Purple Heart, and then was denied all disability and medical benefits on the grounds that his headaches and hearing loss were not caused by the 107mm rocket that knocked him unconscious, but instead by a pre-existing personality disorder.

Soldiers discharged with personality disorders are denied the opportunity to see a medical board and receive a disability rating, so they enter into a bureaucratic no-man's land. And that happened to Town. He submitted an application for VA medical care shortly before leaving the Army, but still was waiting for an appointment seven months later. Without treatment, he struggled alone with deafness, memory loss, sleeplessness, and raging headaches. He couldn't hold a job due to his medical problems, and his wife Kristy had to keep the family of four afloat with her minimum-wage job on an assembly line in Ohio. Soon the family was close to bankruptcy, and the phone company shut off service due to unpaid bills. Then came *The Nation* cover story, followed by an episode of "Law and Order" that introduced his tragedy to nine million viewers. One reader was rock musician Dave Matthews, who began organizing fundraisers and a petition drive.

"There are times when an injustice is so clear that it's not a matter of opinion," said Matthews. "Nobody would argue that what is happening to Jon Town is right. And to think it's happening over and over again… it's just astounding. It's a crime against these young people that's so profound — and it's happening right now."

That stirred another story by the Findley *Courier*, Town's hometown newspaper, which caught the eye of an admiral who works for the VA. He flagged the case, and Town finally won a 100 percent disability rating. By this time, the case had received so much publicity that Rep. Bob Filner invited Town to testify before the House VA Committee, which he chairs. Town told the committee: "I want to state that I did not have a personality disorder before I went into the Army, as they have stated in my paperwork. I did not suffer severe nonstop headaches. I did not have memory loss. I did not have endless, sleepless nights. I have post-traumatic stress disorder and traumatic brain injury now due to the injuries I received in the war, for which I received a Purple Heart. I shouldn't be labeled for the rest of my life with a personality disorder, and neither should my fellow soldiers who also incorrectly received this stigma."

The Nation had already written that the Army's acting surgeon general, Maj. Gen. Gale Pollock, had said that her office had "thoughtfully and thoroughly" reviewed all the cases of personality disorder, including Town's, and had found that each diagnosis was justified. But *The Nation* reported that Pollock's office had not bothered to interview anyone, not even the soldiers whose cases they were supposedly reviewing. Later, the Army conceded that it was unable to even find some of the case files. Furthermore, the "review" was done by the same doctor who had delivered the original diagnosis, Col. Steven Knorr, chief of the Fort Carson Behavioral Health unit! Knorr told the *Army Times* that there was a simple reason why so many cases of underlying personality disorder were being diagnosed among combat troops who had shown no earlier symptoms. Traumatic experiences can trigger a condition that has lain dormant for years, he asserted. "[Troops] may have done fine in high school and before, but it comes out during the stress of service," he said. That assertion was a sharp break from accepted medical procedure, and it triggered angry responses from PTSD counselors and leaders of vet groups.

Filner invited Pollock to testify before his congressional committee after Town had finished, but she sent a subordinate, Col. Bruce Crow, to the stand and take the heat. Crow told the congressman that Pollock would review the cases of 295 personality discharge cases, assisted by "a team of senior mental health providers."

But Rep. Filner would have none of it. He said the allegation "that there's a systematic and policy-driven misdiagnosis of PTSD as personality disorder to get rid of soldiers early, to prevent any expenditures in the future, which were calculated in the billions of dollars … it's a pretty serious allegation. And if you think we're going to believe an evaluation of 295 cases, whichever ones you happen to pick — that we're going to believe what you say — I'll tell you now, I'm not going to believe it. So why bother? Let's have an independent evaluation."

So far, that independent evaluation has been largely in the press. *The Nation* concluded: "Further investigation by *The Nation* has uncovered more than a dozen cases like Town's from bases across the country. All the soldiers interviewed passed the rigorous health screening given recruits before being accepted into the Army. All were deemed physically and psychologically fit in a second screening as well, before being deployed to Iraq where they served honorably in combat. None of the soldiers interviewed during this 11-month investigation had a documented history of psychological problems. Yet after they returned from Iraq, wounded and seeking treatment, each was diagnosed with a pre-existing personality disorder, then denied benefits. As in Town's case, Army doctors determined that the soldiers' ailments were pre-existing without interviewing friends, family, or fellow soldiers who knew them before they were wounded in combat."

That's simply outrageous, and the public needs to know how some of our soldiers are being treated. Again, it's a way of holding callous and indifferent bureaucrats accountable for what they do.

- 15 -
VA: overload and confusion

The VA helps a lot of people, but the vets say you have to fight hard to win their services. It's a bureaucracy that's underfunded, overworked, and mired in red tape — in many ways a mirror image of the Army it was designed to provide service after.

It's not perfect, but the Montana Veterans Affairs Health Care System gets relatively high marks from some disabled combat vets. "I have nothing but good things to say about the VA in Montana," said Laurence Kiefer, Jr. of Bigfork, a former soldier who was medevacced out of Iraq four years ago.

Kiefer told me he was seriously injured as he escorted a semi driven by an Iraqi who was supposed to be delivering a load of food to the commissary on the Tillil military base south of Baghdad. "After the driver blew through the MP [military police] station, I charged my weapon," Kiefer said. "He was trying to get through the gate, so I shot him in the head and he rolled the semi. I damn near went through the windshield."

Kiefer said he had problems with the care at the Walter Reed Medical Center and at Fort Carson, Colorado where he was treated for head injuries and post-traumatic stress disorder. "But Montana has the best VA in the country, according to my [service] brothers around the country," he said. "I tell them that the VA is doing this and this and this for me, and they tell me they aren't getting that kind of help outside of Montana."

Montana does things differently

But an examination of the VA's national database by McClatchy Newspapers suggests otherwise. The newspaper chain filed Freedom of Information Act requests for all three million VA disability claims nationally and the 77 million medical appointments in the agency's health system during 2006. It found the Montana VA offered less specialized mental health care than most other states. Veterans seeking to enter the VA's hospital at Fort Harrison had longer waits and received fewer medical appointments than in almost any other VA hospital in the country.

VA records showed that the Montana VA was spending only six percent of its budget on mental health treatment, ranking 123rd among 138 facilities. Top ranked were White City, Oregon (58 percent); Coatesville, Pennsylvania (44 percent); and Northampton, Maine (40 percent). It also showed that Montana ranked next to last in the percentage of vets with mental illness who received some treatment from VA mental health specialists. In Montana, 55 percent of the vets received some treatment, ranking 137th. The top three facilities — Canandaigua, New York; Poplar Bluff, Missouri; and Albany, New York — all treated 100 percent of the mentally ill vets.

While the average veteran receiving specialized mental health care treatment received 11 visits a year, those who used the Helena hospital and its related clinics received an average of 4.2 visits a year, dead last in the nation. And Fort Harrison was third to last in treating mental illness promptly. While the VA seeks to get vets in to see a doctor within 30 days of their first request for help, that only happened 53 percent of the time in Montana during 2006, according to McClatchy.

Furthermore, the VA's Rocky Mountain Region, which includes Montana. Wyoming, Utah, and Colorado, was in the bottom half of the nation's 21 VA regions, McClatchy found. In a measurement of treatment effectiveness, in which researchers charted patients' progress by comparing pre-treatment and post-treatment mental health scores, the region ranked last.

However, state VA officials defend their system, saying McClatchy didn't understand that Montana's size and its low population density force the VA to operate differently here. "Montana is the only state in the nation that uses private mental health providers," said Joe Underkofler, director of the Veterans Administration Health Care System. "I never want to hear that a vet in crisis has to drive past Benefis Healthcare (about 100 miles north in Great Falls) to get to Fort Harrison for treatment. And if Benefis feels a vet needs more care, we'll send them directly down to Fort Sheridan, Wyoming, without reporting here. That cuts one visit, but it saves time and expense."

McClatchy newspaper reports didn't take into account the state's private contract providers, he said. In 2007, the Montana VA spent $1.8 million on private mental health care providers.

"That report really surprised me," said Sgt. 1st Class Calvin James of the 163rd Infantry Battalion in Helena. "The VA has been of more help to me than any other organization I've dealt with in Montana."

Underkofler said a geographic boundary skewed the statistics presented by McClatchy newspapers. Montana VA doesn't have its own psych ward so it sends many acute PTSD patients to Fort Sheridan, about 100 miles south of Billings. And when the general VA hospital outside Helena is compared with a specialized psych ward, "It's comparing apples and oranges," Underkofler said. The VA said it sent 115 vets from Montana to Fort Sheridan in the 13-month period from July 2006 to August 2007, including 45 Vietnam vets, 23 post-Vietnam vets, 35 Persian Gulf, five Gulf War, three Operation Iraqi Freedom, and two each from Korea and World War II. "All of these were moved either the same day or the next day," said VA information officer Teresa Bell. "Most were moved the same day they were seen as walk-ins."

Private contractors also explain why Montana appears to spend so little of its budget on mental health care, said Underkofler. He said the VA has contracts with hospitals in Billings and Missoula, as well as the Mental Health Center in Great Falls, which has 12 regional clinics. The Western Montana Mental Health Center has 13 regional clinics, while South Central Mental Health has four offices, but subcontracts with Eastern Montana, which has nine other offices based around Miles City. "They provide mental health counseling in their communities of residence," explained Underkofler. "Last year, more than 26,000 mental health visits occurred in the private sector. We've been very successful in using private providers."

He said the number of VA mental health care contract visits has increased from 3,881 in 2003 to more than 22,000 in 2007. With more than 2,000 vets seeking help last year, that averages out to 11 visits each to a contracted clinician. The VA also pays for treatment by private psychologists in rural areas where no clinic service is available.

In fiscal year 2007, Fort Harrison spent 20.2 percent of its budget on mental health care treatment, including its private contract services, said Bell. And in the last quarter of 2007, 94.2 percent of the 324 new patients were able to get an appointment within 30 days, she said, while 95.5 percent of the 2,389 established patients were able to get an appointment within 30 days.

Finally, 2006 was a tough year for the VA at Fort Harrison because it was engulfed by the return of about 700 members of the Montana National Guard's 163rd Infantry Battalion, the largest deployment of troops from the state since World War II. The troops returned home at the end of October 2005.

"The impact of the 163rd was more than just their numbers," said Underkofler. "When the 163rd returned, we discovered people needed help for more than just the obvious injuries. That's when the military began to realize the magnitude of PTSD and TBI. We began to see more hidden injuries."

Phay Lloyd, the VA's OEF/OIF program manager at Fort Harrison, said 185 of the state's 2,055 enrolled Iraqi vets had tested positive for traumatic brain injury as of December 31, 2007.

As to the effectiveness of treatment, Underkofler said that would be impossible to assess since all cases are so markedly different. "We're frankly baffled by where they drew that conclusion. There's nothing we know that measures effectiveness of treatment comparatively, facility by facility. That would be a very subjective evaluation." Some cases of PTSD can never be cured, he said, and life provides different challenges for each traumatized vet. "No program can control life issues," he explained. "We can only teach people to cope with them. But if they have a midlife crisis or a death in the family and begin to run into problems again, is that the fault of the program?"

Despite McClatchy's report, a number of Montana vets say the VA has provided good mental health care. "In the year that I've been here, I've never heard of one of our vets who was unable to get an appointment," said Lucinda Leon, case manager for the Cruse Home, a transitional center that houses up to 11 homeless vets in Helena. "And I've personally had outstanding care there," she added. "I've been there for medical and for mental health care, and they've been outstanding."

No faith in military recordkeeping

Four years after his injury, Laurence Kiefer is still plagued by the effects of PTSD. "I go to bed every night at 9, but I don't get any more than about three hours of sleep," he said. "I'm still waking up with nightmares, and I go through two or three anxiety attacks a day. And when I'm in a store, I don't like to have anyone standing behind me."

Kiefer doesn't trust the system at all. He insists on documenting every aspect of his care because he said the Army is notorious for losing records. He also reads extensively about his symptoms and second-guesses his military doctors when he thinks they're wrong in their diagnosis or treatment.

"They gave me a less-than-honorable discharge, which ruined my dental and health care benefits," he said. "Basically, it means you get no benefits. I had to hire an attorney to fight for an honorable discharge, and we managed to get it corrected. They said it was a typo, but they did it to me deliberately because they knew I was a troublemaker. It's really sad that they have that kind of power."

Dr. James Peake, the VA secretary, can't believe such abuses of power. "This agency is absolutely dedicated to doing the best job we can for our veterans, but some of our protocols date back to 1945 and need to be modernized. Particularly, our paper process needs to become updated," he told me.

Mission to help vets

With fewer than a million residents, Montana has about 108,000 veterans, putting it among the highest number of vets per capita, said Underkofler. About 5,000 of those are Iraq/Afghanistan vets, and 1,500 of them are currently receiving medical services, he said. That puts Montana almost on par with the national estimate that about one in four returning soldiers will be treated for emotional disorders, including post-traumatic stress disorder and traumatic brain injury.

With the increasing workload, the VA medical center has been gearing up. "In the past two years, the resources have been much more forthcoming and our budgets have been healthy," Underkofler said. "We've added about 15 staffers to this facility due to increased funding and a mental-health emphasis. We're about to commit to a third psychiatrist — we never had three psychiatrists before."

But it's not easy to recruit physicians to a non-metropolitan state like Montana, said Dr. Rosa Merino, chief of psychiatry for the VA Montana Health Care Systems. "We got a PTSD grant that provided for three positions, but we've been trying to recruit two psychologists for more than a year."

Outlying programs are particularly important in places like Montana's Daniels County, where not much help is available, said Vera Lynn Trangsrud of Scobey, who's active in an organization called Daniels County Military Families.

The group came together several years ago to assemble care packages for a number of service members serving in Iraq and Afghanistan, something it continues to do for half a dozen soldiers still deployed. But it's evolving into a support group for families struggling with the aftermath of serving in the war, Trangsrud said.

She agonizes over her son in Billings, who is fighting PTSD, depression, and thoughts of suicide. "I have a total feeling of hopelessness. You want to reach out, but nothing you say makes them feel any better. I've never in my life experienced such a feeling of helplessness," she added. She's hoping that the VA will set up an outpost in Wolf Point to help veterans and their families in northeastern Montana. "I think families need support groups as much as the vets do," she said.

Independent investigation requested

The McClatchy report prompted Montana's two U.S. senators, Max Baucus and Jon Tester, to ask the VA to investigate its operations in Montana and determine how the system could be improved.

That request for an investigation went directly to the agency's inspector general, who is examining the situation, said Dr. Peake, the secretary of Veterans Affairs. "Unfortunately, the newspaper underestimated by about half the amount we spend on mental health care in Montana," Peake told me. "Due to the unique nature of Montana, we spend about as much externally [on outside contractors] as we do internally. So that report underestimates our services in Montana by about half."

Frustration and failure

For some high-strung soldiers, though, the VA bureaucracy can be too much.

"I gave up on them," said Jeremiah Thompson of Billings, a retired Marine who later joined a private military group as a private security contractor. "I tried to fill out the paperwork to register, but they changed the form and sent it back to me. At the time, I was having a lot of problems, anxiety and depression, and I got so frustrated I gave up."

When Thompson explained his plight to the Montana Post-Deployment Health Reassessment Task Force in Helena, Eric Kettenring of the Missoula Vet Center had a quick suggestion. "Every vet can go to the Vet Center for free, and for life," Kettenring told him.

"But it's overloaded," Thompson responded. "You don't get help because they're so swamped." Thompson later said that a bigger problem was his private security work. "The Vet Center has a book that tells them if you've seen enough incidents to qualify for post-traumatic," he said. "In the Marine Corps, I didn't qualify. In the private sector, I was more than qualified. But that wasn't their problem."

Thompson won't say which private security firm he was working for, but he said he saw more combat with them than he did as a Marine deployed all over the globe. "The first incident was when an IED exploded in the vehicle in front of me," he said. "One gentleman passed away, another was severely wounded in the stomach, and another took shrapnel in the jaw. It's not pleasant to see someone die in front of you. Then a friend of mine was shot in the head by a sniper in a firefight. He died in the tower, and I had to carry him out. On another occasion, a rocket exploded about 50 yards from me. I was fine, but shrapnel killed a Marine. He was bleeding out and I was first on the scene to administer first aid, trying to stop the bleeding, trying to keep him breathing, but he died. He had no pulse."

When he left Iraq, Thompson knew he had a problem. "When I first got back, I couldn't sleep in a bed," he said. "I slept on the floor with a gun, and I had anxiety nightmares." With the Vet Center out of the picture and his refusal to tolerate the VA paperwork, Thompson tried to find help in the private sector, but found counselors just as busy. "Just to get in the door and talk with someone takes six months," Thompson said. "And I was told by some that workers' compensation is not an acceptable form of payment." Finally a private psychologist, Tim Richter, took Thompson on as a patient, and they hit it off together. Today, Thompson said he can see improvement to the point where he and Richter would like to put together a vets' support group.

But the issue of caring for the emotional disorders of private security contractors must be addressed because the Pentagon said one in four combatants working for the federal government in Iraq is a private security contractor. They'll be among the highest-stressed vets that will be returning. And while they made excellent money overseas, it's unlikely they'll have a disability package funded by their private employers. So they're going to need help. And if they don't get it, we all will pay. Since the private contractors were working for the Department of Defense, the VA needs to find a way to assist them.

Combat mental triage

Underkofler agrees that vets like Thompson would be better advised to seek help from the VA. "The VA hospital deals with all vets, while the Vet Center deals with combat vets," he said. Montana has Vet Centers in Missoula and Billings that are generally staffed by combat vets who help other vets.

At a meeting of the Montana Post-Deployment Health Reassessment Task Force in Helena, a number of people worried about vets falling through the cracks. Some suggested that counseling ought to be mandatory for the first year or two after a veteran returns from combat.

"That's illegal," responded Underkofler. "Just because someone has been in Iraq, you can't say he has to go to treatment. And it won't work. Treatment only works when you seek it out because you know you need it."

A group of vets is working with the VA to provide an informal network of veterans to work with others who are returning and readjusting. It's a program called Vet-to-Vet.

"We'd be happy to sit down with any vet, have coffee and help them," said Tom Huddleston of Helena, a disabled Vietnam vet with PTSD. Chapters have started in Great Falls, Missoula, and Bozeman.

"We welcome any vet who wants to join us," agreed Jerry Burback, co-facilitator of the group in Great Falls. "And if a spouse wants to sit in, he or she is more than welcome. We want to work with the families."

It's a program that Dr. Merino is enthused about. "This program is unique," she said. "It's all about the camaraderie of helping each other, which is what vets are all about. And while helping others, you also help yourself. So it shifts the whole paradigm."

However, the VA will need to have specialized assistance programs in place for women. Nationally, there are currently about 1.7 million female vets, of whom 235,000 are receiving health care from the VA. The number of women seeking treatment can be expected to double within the next five years.

Independent Review

Unfortunately, the VA is blamed for the armed forces' inability to take care of its own active-duty members. Military doctors are largely failing to treat mental disorders among soldiers returning from combat, according to an independent report commissioned by the Department of Defense in the wake of the Walter Reed scandal in 2007. It quoted the American Psychiatric Association as saying, "Our work group has found the consequences of the Iraq and Afghanistan wars to be a national public health crisis."

The report also found that although military medical needs skyrocketed because of returning disabled soldiers, DOD spending didn't even keep pace with the civilian medical inflation. It also recommended establishing a medical treatment and research center devoted solely to brain injuries. Barebones military medical funding can't keep up with the increasing caseload, the review group concluded. It noted that national health expenditures increased by 28.4 percent from 2003 through 2006, but the Walter Reed budget grew by only 12.3 percent.

"This lag in budget growth at these military medical facilities that have been receiving and treating casualties, in comparison to the national health expenditures during this same time period, are questionable," the report stated. Furthermore, funding levels are likely to drop, it found. The group said that the DOD has adopted an accounting measure called the "efficiency wedge," which presumes efficiencies gained by implementing a new payment system, then cuts the budget by that amount. That style of accounting meant Army hospitals lost $30 million in funding for fiscal year 2006 and another $82 million in fiscal year 2007. The acting Army surgeon general told Congress that Army hospitals would have to begin cutting services if they lost $142 million in fiscal year 2008, as projected.

The review board also found that staff is overwhelmed. "In years past, there have been approximately 450 active-duty licensed clinical psychologists serving their country in uniform," the review group said. "Today, that number has shrunk to less than 350 [a 22 percent decrease], and the rate of attrition continues at an alarming rate."

Furthermore, service members returning from combat are denied immediate medical help, the group said. "The Medical Hold and Holdover companies are not properly staffed to provide guidance to patients, especially those with traumatic brain injury and post-traumatic stress disorder," the report stated. "Also, there are no medical personnel on staff to provide care and counseling to patients."

"I spent a year in Medical Hold at Fort Carson and it was a compete farce," said Kiefer of Bigfork. "Their treatment was just to throw more pills at you. I had 43 different medications, and the hydrochloric thiazide gave me gout. They really didn't know how to deal with the wounded." Separation and solitude also were bad for patients, Kiefer said. "I think the plan was to hold you there until you lost your wife. The divorce rate at the time was about 85 percent, and I was one of them."

The review board also expressed a concern that Guard and Reserve soldiers don't receive adequate care. One problem is that some providers don't accept TRICARE, the government's managed health care program. "The volume of documentation and time delay in payment were the leading causes for the providers' reluctance to accept TRICARE," the report states.

Reforms

The review board suggested a number of reforms:

- The U.S. secretary of defense should order regulatory reform to make TRICARE more acceptable to providers.
- The Army chief of staff should boost staffing levels for the Medical Hold companies, and the surgeon general should ensure that behavioral specialists are assigned to them.
- The defense secretary should reconsider the "efficiency wedge" during time of war.
- The [DOD] should develop and implement functional and cognitive testing of all recruits entering military service, and veterans leaving it.
- "Exposure to blasts" should be included in each patient's medical record.

- The DOD should develop comprehensive and universal clinical practice guidelines for blast injuries with a PTSD overlay. "This is an urgent requirement," the report states.
- The secretary of defense must urgently review Traumatic Servicemembers' Group Life Insurance to ensure that coverage is expanded to include the full spectrum of traumatic brain injury and post-traumatic stress disorder.
- DOD should establish "a center for excellence for traumatic brain injury and post-traumatic stress disorder. The center should assist military services in meeting their responsibility to train primary care and specialty providers, case managers, Medical Hold and Holdover staffs, unit commanders, patients, and family members on signs, effects, effective management, and proper documentation of traumatic brain injury and post-traumatic stress disorder."

The review group added that it believes injured veterans deserve specialized medical care. "Generally, the nation must recognize that there is a moral, human, and budgetary cost of war," the report concluded. "When we engage in armed conflict, we must recognize those costs and be prepared to execute on those obligations."

Part 2
The Solutions

Here, we look at ways we can improve our system of health care with changes to existing systems and innovative treatment options.

- 16 -
National Guard reform

From Chris Dana's suicide came the impetus to change the way the Montana National Guard looks after soldiers returning from combat. This chapter looks at how the program started, its success, and its role in creating a statewide program to take better care of our returning veterans. Now all veterans and their families are offered care. The care is improved and the stigma of admitting to a problem has been significantly reduced.

Seven months after Chris Dana's suicide in March 2007, the Montana National Guard had a post-deployment health reassessment plan in place and was beginning to implement it. At a legislative hearing in Helena, Montana, Adjutant General Randy Mosley promised that the National Guard would do a better job evaluating the mental health of returning combat vets.

The Montana National Guard had about 2,700 soldiers, 80 percent of whom have deployed to Iraq and Afghanistan.

But Mosley also said that his campaign plan to help combat vets after deployment has no immediate funding because it goes beyond Department of Defense requirements. "It's essential the DOD policies get changed," Mosley told the state legislature's Administration and Veterans Affairs Interim Committee. "I can augment and supplement, but that means I have to find the funding to do it."

And that's a statement that has broad national ramifications. The federal government must adopt similar solutions to make sure they're available to all soldiers, across the board, whether they came from units in Montana or Mississippi.

Mosley said he has sent funding requests to the National Guard Bureau, his national organization, and asked for help from Montana's congressional delegation. "And I will bring to your attention areas in which the federal government is unwilling to support my efforts in the hopes you may help me take the actions that Montanans require," Mosley told legislators.

Mosley said it was wrong that no one knew that Dana had been suffering from PTSD.

"We started discharging people, in some cases without realizing that they had medical or mental health reasons for not attending their drills," Mosley said. "I have directed that we will not issue any more less-than-honorable discharges unless I personally review the case and approve it."

Mosley endorsed all 10 problem areas and 14 specific solutions suggested by the task force, "and we will implement them — and more." He promised that the National Guard will create a pilot crisis response team to investigate cases in which soldiers begin falling away from their drill duties. It will consist of a chaplain, a career counselor, and a command sergeant major or chief master sergeant from outside the soldier's normal chain of command.

All soldiers leaving the service will receive a mental health evaluation before they leave, he said. "We will do mental health assessments four times on all our soldiers over the first two years post deployment and every year thereafter for as long as they remain in the Guard," said Mosley.

Task Force Recommendations

These were the recommendations that the Post Deployment Health Reassessment Task Force made for the Montana National Guard.

1. Evaluate medical status before discharge
2. Allow Guardsmen to request honorable discharge
3. Thoroughly review all Guard PDHRA personnel files for completion
4. Expand the PDHRA process
5. Mandate enrollment in the VA health care system
6. Present awards and medals to Guardsmen within 90 days
7. Send badge information to DOD within 90 days
8. Include mental health focus in training
9. Increase awareness of available resources
10. Create Crisis Response Team
11. Allow drill attendance upon return home
12. Increase informal support systems — Vet-to-Vet
13. Enhance Family Readiness Program
14. Form partnership with State Veterans Groups

He said he has requested funding for the additional testing, but had no idea what it might cost. "We don't have a single mental health professional attached to headquarters, and that's unacceptable to me," he added. "So we'll have to get funding for that, too."

Mosley said it's obviously a mistake to give National Guardsmen 90 days off all military duty after returning from combat because it isolates them by removing one important support group [service buddies]. "Since DOD does not require drills during that 90-day period, they took the money away to pay our soldiers for attending drills," Mosley told legislators. "Right now, Defense Secretary Robert Gates has granted a one-state policy exemption as a pilot program to Minnesota, and I've asked that Montana be included in that exemption," he said.

Another recommendation the National Guard will implement is to strengthen the family readiness programs. "The sad fact is that the family readiness unit funding is based on the number of people deployed, and when the soldiers come home, that funding disappears," Mosley said.

"But the vets and their families have told us that they continue to need that support after they return home, so I've asked DOD and our congressional delegation for help in getting the additional funding."

Chris Dana's stepbrother Matt Kuntz told state legislators at the hearing that the federal government, not the state Legislature, should be forced to pick up the tab. "With all due respect, senators and representatives, you did not vote for this war. The federal government did. We merely provided the troops. So they should be required to pay for the damage they did to them. If this was a private company that came in and damaged the mental health of its employees in Montana, they'd be required to correct those problems. I believe the federal government should be required to do the same."

Kuntz applauded the additional mental health evaluations. "You need to expect that the people who have been put into combat will come back with PTSD," he said. "I think we need a system that expects those people to have PTSD and requires them to prove they don't have it."

Ron Skinner of the Valley Veterans Service Center in Hamilton praised the campaign plan, although he said there should be no time limit on mental health assessments. "I'm a Vietnam vet, 1967-68, but it wasn't until 1980 that I walked into a counselor's office and said, 'I hope you have a rubber room because I need it.' So I'm concerned about a two-year time frame for evaluations. I think that's a big hole."

Tracy Velazquez, executive director of the Montana Mental Health Association, commended the campaign plan, adding, "It's clear they've gone the extra mile."

"I've read this report, and it's an amazing document," agreed Kuntz. "I was a bitter guy [after his stepbrother's suicide], but I'm a believer now because this group got it. And I'm proud to know that Adjutant General Mosley has already begun to implement parts of this plan."

After the meeting, Randy Mosley said the National Guard would implement the plan fully — one way or another. "Right now, there isn't the money to do any of the things we're promising, so I'll have to ask Montanans to provide the community support to raise this money."

Noting that it's been only seven months since Dana's suicide, he called the campaign plan a work in progress. Now that they know what's needed, the next step will be to determine costs. "I don't want to pull a number out of the air," he said. "I'm sure it's a million dollars, probably several."

One reason for the higher figure — and for the uncertainty — is that the task force wisely expanded the need for treatment to all veterans statewide, not just those coming home from Iraq and Afghanistan.

"Montana National Guard combat veterans are but a microcosm of those who reside in our large state, which include those still serving, those discharged from their Guard or Reserve units, and those discharged from active military service," it said. "Recommendations in this report envision a statewide network of education, support services, and resources that will meaningfully assist Montana's veterans to cope with the emotional and mental health issues resulting from serving in combat and who — once home — are expected to smoothly reintegrate into a civilian lifestyle."

No shortage of new recruits

Despite the potential danger of facing combat, the Montana National Guard has been remarkably successful in enlisting new recruits.

"If you're taking care of soldiers and their families, they're walking billboards for you," said Maj. Barry Gilman, chief of recruiting and retention for the Montana National Guard.

The national goal is to keep attrition rates below 18 percent, but Montana's is at 13.9 percent for fiscal 2008, the eighth best in the nation, Gilman said. In 2007, the National Guard had 518 new enlistees, including 363 with no prior military experience and 155 veterans. "That brought our troop strength up to just below 2,700 soldiers," said Gilman. "The last time we were at those levels was 1997, so that's our baseline."

One big reason for the success is a "Bring your buddy to drill" campaign in which current soldiers get a $2,000 bonus for each recruit who signs up. "We've already paid out right at $700,000 in the state of Montana," Gilman said. "Not only is this money that stays in the state economy, but it's money that goes directly into soldiers' pockets."

Logan Krause, a senior at Fort Benton High School who's carrying a 3.85 grade point average, is taking advantage of the Guard Recruiting Assistance Program. "I wasn't GRAPed myself," he said, "but I was able to recruit one of my high school buddies." Krause signed up for training to become a National Guard firefighter after he graduates from high school. "Sense of duty was the main reason I signed up, but the college benefits can't be argued with," Krause said. "In fact, all the benefits were huge."

Sgt. 1st Class Rick Haerter, the National Guard's recruiter in Great Falls, said GRAP goes well beyond the financial incentive, however. "The biggest thing is that they get to be around people like themselves, people who like the military and want to join it," Haerter said. "About 80 percent of the time, these kids tell me that the biggest thing for them is service to their country."

At the Centerville High School, Haerter dropped in to visit with a couple of students who had recently enlisted. "College benefits are part of it, but there's a military background in my family that I want to continue," said senior Courtney Martin, who has a 4.0 GPA and is planning to become a military medic. Her dad spent 20 years with the Air National Guard after a stint in the active-duty Air Force, she explained. And junior Justin Basaraba said, "I want to use this as a stepping stone to join the Special Forces."

Haerter has signed up 20 kids in a five-month period despite a directive that four Guard units, including the 163rd Armored Cavalry Regiment based in Belgrade, begin increased training for a probable deployment to Iraq in the next year or two. Most soldiers expect a new deployment and accept it, said Haerter, who is also retention officer for his company of the 163rd. "We lost a few guys [after the last deployment in 2004-05], but not very many," he said. "They just decided it was time to do something different. Over the past year, we've only had two soldiers who ETSed [terminated service]. The rest have re-enlisted."

While in Iraq, the 163rd saw moderate to heavy combat, doing house-to-house searches while being bombarded regularly with mortars and rocked by roadside bombs. Two Montana soldiers were killed there, and another came home to Cascade paralyzed from the waist down by a sniper.

Gilman said the 163rd returned from Iraq with an authorized strength of 725 soldiers and immediately reorganized into a heavy combat arms battalion utilizing Bradley tanks. "Its assigned strength today is now 848 personnel," he said. "It has 925 soldiers and it's at 109 percent of its assigned strength. That's currently the highest-strength battalion in the state."

Another key has been that the National Guard has assigned senior non-commissioned officers (NCOs) to serve as career counselors in each of Montana's four battalions, listening to and addressing concerns of the soldiers and their families, Gilman said. "What we've been doing in terms of family support groups has been of tremendous value in retaining our soldiers."

Not everyone concurs with that upbeat assessment

"I don't have much good to say about them. I figure that a lot of that touchy-feely, feel-good stuff is bullshit," says Doug Casson, a former firefighter and first responder for the Montana Air National Guard. "When they found out I had PTSD, they pretty well marched me out the door. They couldn't get rid of me fast enough."

Casson concedes, however, that he gave them cause when he blew up and threatened to kill them all in one ill-considered moment.

Casson blames his problems on spending four months of 2004 in Iraq when he was in charge of firefighter/emergency medical technician crews, dealing personally with the dead or wounded and directing 33 subordinates into situations where they might be killed. "We were attacked regularly, but we also had medical emergencies," he said. "We had one guy run over by a deuce-and-a-half [truck], and he was popped like a zit."

In Iraq, Casson said he was credited with surviving more than 100 enemy attacks at Forward Operating Base Anaconda (also known as Balad), but he said they took their toll. "The second week, we had a mortar blow up 50 feet from our fire rescue truck," he said. "It was close enough that we could see smoke blowing out of the air-conditioning ducts. The impact was so great that we couldn't see or hear — our only sense was touch. When our senses finally returned, we realized that none of us were wounded, that we were walking away from it."

The concussion may have contributed to a later bout of diverticulitis, he said, but he was never tested for traumatic brain injury.

The base was attacked three or four times a day, including one day in which a medevac chopper and the medevac tent were hit. Casson's unit was first on the scene. "Twenty medics were there, but they weren't doing anything because they were in shock. One flight medic had a chunk of wood the size of a broom handle go through her breast right below the nipple and into her chest."

Another major attack on the base he has blocked out. "I just remember that we had 200 to 300 people standing in line to give blood, and each bag of blood went directly to a wounded soldier," he said.

Another attack focused on the base exchange (BX), a direct hit that made Casson suspect that Iraqis working on the base in the daytime went back to the insurgents at night and helped them hit areas with the greatest number of targets. "They'd usually try to hit the chow line at breakfast, lunch, and dinner to get the greatest number of casualties. It made you not want to be spending much time in the mess hall." But the first responders weren't there much anyway. "When the first rocket hits, while people are running for their shelters, our rescue units get rolling," he said. "It gets pretty chaotic to try to decide where to go and still stay alive."

The base exchange attack killed four or five soldiers and wounded another 32, he said. "One guy who was killed had been going home and he had been given an hour to go the BX to get a souvenir for his kid. I watched an officer bleed to death when his jugular was hit by a fragment as he was trying to help one of his wounded men. It was hard to see these 18-year-olds and 19-year-olds getting killed."

He also remembers a C-141 touching down on the base airstrip, loading up wounded soldiers for further treatment at a military hospital in Germany. As his rescue unit headed out to the plane, mortars began to fall on the tarmac. "We jumped out of the fire truck and began offloading those stretchers [to take the wounded to the C-141] right in the midst of all those incoming mortars," he said. "The higher-ups from that unit told me we should have gotten the Bronze Star for heroism under fire, but instead we got reprimanded for leaving the fire truck."

Coming home was a surreal experience. Friends held a party to celebrate. "But we only stayed about 15 minutes. The kids all had balloons and were popping them. When we dropped to our knees, everybody thought that was pretty funny, so we left."

For a year, Casson said he realized he was having increasingly severe problems, but he hid them. "I had trouble sleeping because the dead were haunting me in my sleep," he said. "The Guard didn't have any programs for PTSD so I began going to a private psychologist."

Then the diverticulitis kicked in again, and he underwent surgery to relieve it and his acid reflux problem. When he came back, he had medical appointments, but he said his superiors accused him of malingering and faking the symptoms of PTSD. They'd also promised him a promotion, but gave it instead to a youngster with a third of his experience who had been filling in for him while he was ill.

At that point, he blew it. "I told them I was seeing a shrink and taking meds so I didn't kill all you motherfuckers," he said.

He went home to cool off, but when he went back on base the next day, he said he was spread-eagled and searched. Then he was barred from the base where he'd been a fire department supervisor, allowed entry only with special permission. For a year, he was in limbo and without income. "I didn't know how we were going to make it," he said. "We were looking at selling the house and the cars just to be able to survive."

Finally, the active-duty doctors concluded he had severe PTSD and awarded him a 50 percent disability in November 2006. "On that final day, I didn't do any of the normal outprocessing," Casson said. "Instead, they brought the paperwork out to the gate and I signed it there. No one at the Air National Guard helped me."

Officials of the Air National Guard dispute most of Casson's story. His commanding officer, Lt. Col. Corey Halvorson, said he can't find any record of a medevac chopper being hit on the tarmac, the chow line being mortared, or a line of soldiers waiting to give blood. The BX did get hit, but Halvorson said Casson's unit was not one of the responders. And the chunk of wood the size of a broom handle in the flight medic's breast was a sliver that was removed with a needle and tweezers.

"Through my prior investigation interviews with his coworkers and supervisors there in Iraq, very few mortars landed within his sector and most were duds," said Halvorson. "I have never heard of any certificates of my men 'surviving enemy attacks,' His peers did not receive such recognition and I have never heard of such recognition within our armed forces."

But Casson has a certificate that names him and reads, "I survived 100 attacks at Balad AB Iraq." And he has letters from two co-workers that were submitted to the VA to substantiate his claim for disability benefits. One of them said, "TSGT Casson manned the rescue truck 24/7 and never had a break. He ran on all calls to station 1. By the time the department was fully staffed, he was looking exhausted both physically and mentally. He was my station captain and lead rescue man on the rescue truck. His job on the rescue truck was to respond to all emergencies to include: aircraft in-flight emergencies, structural fires, vehicle fires, and medical emergencies. We were attacked every day by rockets and mortars."

Another co-worker wrote: "During our time in Balad, we were attacked every day. I remember once when he was responding to an attack, he was almost killed by a rocket that landed by his rescue truck. That shook him up. Another time his bunkroom was nicked by an incoming rocket. While he was sleeping beside the wall, the rocket hit, the fins of the rocket left scratch marks on the outside of his wall. He stated that scared the hell out of him. He responded to many attacks that had wounded. One time he responded to a direct hit at the army medevac squadron. The hit was directly on their sleeping quarters. He had five wounded, three were critical, and two were minor injuries. Another time he had to respond to a direct hit by a mortar at the main BX. He had 30 wounded from life threatening to minor injuries, plus three or four were confirmed dead."

What can we believe in this troubling story and the equally troubling official denial? A couple of things stand out clearly to me. First, Casson was in a combat zone and, despite the testimony of his commanding officer, underwent considerable trauma. Second, he came back with emotional disorders that were ultimately diagnosed as PTSD. Third, as a result of that disorder, he is filled with a tremendous amount of anger, which pushes away the people who ought to be coming forward to get him help. That continues today. He's still barred from the base without a security escort.

"Instead of getting him help, the Guard only tried to push him out," said his wife, Tina. Casson added, "Then the VA came in and bent over backward to help me. They get a bad name sometimes, but the VA saved my life."

When Chris Dana killed himself, Casson didn't immediately recognize it as a turning point. But he does now. "That was what it took — one guy blowing his brains out — to change the system. But it's too late for a lot of guys like me. The Air National Guard is convinced I'm taking advantage of the system. They set out to destroy me, and they nearly succeeded."

Larry Seibel, wing command chief for the Montana Air National Guard's 120th Fighter Wing in Great Falls, can't discuss specific cases, but said things have changed. "A commander's job is to protect the base so a soldier who makes a threat might be barred from the base, might be allowed on base only with an escort, and would probably be relieved from his military job where he might pose a threat." But, he added, the first order of business now would be to get help for a soldier suffering from PTSD.

As you have seen throughout this book, there are still thousands of other vets who continue to suffer, many of them in silence.

Montana becomes a national pilot program

Eleven months after Chris Dana's suicide, the Montana National Guard was selected to start a national pilot program to perform additional mental health screenings on military veterans returning from service overseas. The additional screenings will help more quickly detect mental health problems such as post-traumatic stress disorder, so military personnel can more effectively and efficiently get the treatment they need, Senators Max Baucus and Jon Tester said.

"I'm really happy," said Kuntz, Dana's stepbrother. "This is a huge testament to how far Montana and its politicians have come in the past year."

Baucus and Tester met with Under Secretary of Defense for Personnel and Readiness, Dr. David Chu, in December 2007 and urged the National Guard to provide a second mental health screening for troops returning from combat after they had time to settle back into life in Montana. The senators said that Montana is the only state in the country that will conduct the additional screenings. The National Guard will use the state as a pilot program to determine the effectiveness of the second screenings. If the program is successful, the National Guard will make the additional screenings available in other states as well.

"No one understands the importance of Montana's people becoming involved and calling the governor [Brian Schweitzer] and telling him to fix this problem," said Kuntz. "He jumped on it, the National Guard got on board, and senators Baucus and Tester made sure the funding came through." That's how democracy is supposed to work, Kuntz said.

The screenings, which the Montana National Guard will conduct during the second year after a deployment for those remaining in the service, will be in addition to one that troops receive right after returning home. Those who serve and leave the military are eligible for Veterans Affairs benefits.

"This is a great day for Montana and an even greater day for our National Guard soldiers and airmen," said Col. Jeff Ireland, director of manpower and personnel for the National Guard in Helena. "We've been really blessed by being given the opportunity to meet the recommendations of our post-deployment task force and the commitment of National Guard commanders." The cost of the additional mental health screening will be paid by the National Guard Bureau, Ireland added.

"Receiving approval for the second Post-Deployment Health Reassessment is a great breakthrough in guardsmen and family care," said Mosley, Montana's adjutant general. "We now have the means to extend this benefit to stay in contact with our soldiers and airmen to ensure they receive the care they deserve. It is of utmost importance to me as commander of the Montana National Guard that our force is taken care of when they come home and transition back to normal life."

Progress after the first anniversary

In the year since the suicide of Chris Dana, the Montana National Guard has put teams in place to get help for other soldiers troubled by post-traumatic stress disorder.

"In my humble opinion, America is facing a huge train wreck due to PTSD," said Larry Seibel of the Montana Air National Guard's 120th Fighter Wing, who heads the crisis response team in Great Falls. "But Montana is in the vanguard of states trying to provide help for soldiers who have come back from their deployments with problems." Today, crisis response teams are in place across the state to help soldiers who seek it or who are referred by their commanders and/or first sergeants.

In Great Falls, the crisis response team has already handled five cases. In January 2008, an airman came to a weekend drill and told her friends that she had slit her wrists due to loneliness and a failing relationship. She was immediately whisked to the Benefis East mental health unit, and then referred to the military sexual trauma unit at Malmstrom Air Force Base near Great Falls for ongoing counseling and treatment, Seibel said. "One of the doctors diagnosed her with PTSD due to the results of a 2004 deployment," he added.

"All the incidents that we have handled have been PTSD-related due to prior deployments," said Nicole Gasvoda, a health technician with the 120th Fighter Wing and a member of the crisis response team. Team members include a senior non-commissioned officer, health professionals, a chaplain, a personnel officer, and the first sergeant and commander of the soldier the team is trying to help.

"We advise the commander of all the tools available to him in our toolbox," Seibel said, adding that those decisions are then made jointly by the commander and the soldier in need of help. "All the people that we've dealt with have sought help." Under a pilot program authorized only in Montana by the National Guard Bureau, the mental health of soldiers is assessed as they leave a theater of combat, then every six months for the next two years, said Jen Fagan, a public health technician for the 120th Fighter Wing.

The first form, the in-theater assessment form, is a seven pager that asks whether a soldier experienced an IED or RPG blast, a vehicle crash, or a wound causing the soldier to lose consciousness, be dazed, unable to remember, suffer a concussion, or a head injury. It asks whether the soldier saw people killed or wounded, discharged a weapon during combat, or felt in great danger of being killed.

"Have you ever had any experience that was so frightening, horrible, or upsetting that IN THE PAST MONTH you: a) have had nightmares about it or thought about it when you did not want to? b) tried hard not to think about it or went out of your way to avoid situations that remind you of it? c) were constantly on guard, watchful, or easily startled? d) felt numb or detached from others, activities, your surroundings?" asks the questionnaire. It also questions exposure to chemicals and there's a section on alcohol use. And it asks whether a soldier would like to see physical health care providers, mental health providers, or a chaplain.

That's followed every six months by an assessment form that asks about the soldier's overall health. It repeats the questions about combat experiences and the questions about nightmares, flashbacks, and alcohol use, adding: "Since your deployment, have you had serious conflicts with your spouse, family members, close friends, or at work that continue to cause you worry or concern?"

"We're the only state in the union to be doing this testing over a two-year period," said Seibel, adding that Mosley has infused the Montana National Guard with a proactive approach toward helping its troops.

Montana becomes a national model

"Montana has gone beyond the level of other states in the country, and I applaud that," said Capt. Joan Hunter, a U.S. Public Service officer who was recently designated director of psychological health for the National Guard Bureau in Washington, DC. "They saw an emergency need, studied the problems, and made some significant improvements."

Adjutant General Mosley acknowledges that this deliberate effort stems from the Guard's earlier failure: Chris Dana, the former soldier who didn't get the help he needed and killed himself a year ago. "We want to make sure we're doing everything we can to help our people and their families pick up the pieces for the problems that may have begun during their deployment in Iraq," Mosley said.

"The Guard has done an unbelievable job in changing," said Kuntz, Dana's stepbrother. "It takes a lot for a big organization that does a lot of things right to look for what they did wrong and address those flaws. I'm really impressed with what they've done."

One of the most important corrections was creating crisis response teams to work with soldiers who are having problems. "Things like the crisis response teams that they started have been very impressive," Hunter said. Another important step was to win permission to exceed Department of Defense guidelines and assess soldiers' mental health every six months for the first two years after deployment.

"So far, our experience has shown us that the problems have begun to show from 18 to 24 months after return from deployment," Mosley said. "So every six months, we want to reach out to our people and check them. And DOD has provided the authorization and funding to provide the additional testing up to two years. To my knowledge, Montana is the only state in the nation to be doing so."

The RAND Corporation recently reported that one in three soldiers returning from deployment in Iraq/Afghanistan suffers from post-traumatic stress disorder, major depression, or minor traumatic brain injury (mTBI). However, the Montana National Guard hasn't yet seen casualties of that magnitude, according to Col. Jeff Ireland. "There is definitely a problem, although we can't determine whether it's PTSD or mTBI." He said it's difficult, though, to gather statistics because some soldiers have endured the problem and persevered while others have sought treatment with private counselors or with the VA. Guardsmen still worry that medical problems can hamper their careers, he notes.

"PTSD is a normal reaction to abnormal circumstances," added Capt. Adam Karlin, deputy state surgeon. "However, the military is beginning to accept that paradigm, and people are willing to accept that they may need help." Karlin also said, however, that the RAND Corporation's one-in-three ratio sounded pretty realistic.

With the additional mental health testing, which is mandatory for all Guardsmen, will come additional personnel. The Guard has added a PDHRA manager, Capt. Jeremy Hedges, as well as two behavioral health specialists. It has also been notified it will join the Joint Family Support

Assistance Program, which will add two military family benefit specialists and one child and youth specialist.

It also expects that the National Guard Bureau will contribute one additional counselor to each state. "In addition to what Montana is doing at the state level, I am in the process of designing a program that will put a director of psychological health in every state," Hunter said. "This individual will be a licensed care provider who will support what Montana has already begun to implement." Hunter said she hopes to have funding for the project in the fiscal year that begins October 1, 2008.

TriWest Healthcare, which is based in Phoenix, has also teamed up with the Montana National Guard to check active-duty soldiers and airmen for symptoms of PTSD. Basing its plan on a pilot program it was already using in California, TriWest is paying to have four part-time behavioral health specialists join the Guard on drill weekends — two at the Montana Air National Guard on Gore Hill in Great Falls and two at the Army National Guard in Fort Harrison outside Helena — to be available to talk with the vets about any problems they may be having. The counselors have already begun to build personal relationships with the Guard personnel, which is a plus. And it makes counseling quick, easy, convenient … and free to the soldier or airman. "Unlike Vietnam, we're not waiting for people to present us with problems," TriWest CEO David McIntyre told me. "We're pushing to get people help as quickly as possible."

For the past two years, TriWest has funded embedded counselors for 37 units of the California National Guard, McIntyre said. Nearly 8,000 encounters with soldiers and airmen in California have yielded 600 referrals for further mental health care. That's a significant improvement, and I'm glad that Montana is beginning to benefit from this program. But it's also clear that this is a program that should be adopted nationwide.

Strengthening Guard families

Combat isn't the only stressor, however. Family problems also contribute. "They may have financial problems or their marriages are going to heck or their kids are out of control," Mosley said. So Montana plans to take advantage of the Beyond the Yellow Ribbon program, recently authorized by the Department of Defense.

"Reintegration has gotten a much stronger focus over the past year," explains Holly Wick, head of the 120th Fighter Wing's Family Readiness Unit. "We're telling families how to reintroduce themselves to each other again and get back on track together."

In New York State, returning Army Guardsmen are required to attend a retreat at an upscale motel — with families invited — first at 30 and again at 60 days after their return from deployment. That allows soldiers to be with their buddies and meet each other's families. It also allows wives to listen in on briefings about family benefits that a combat-focused soldier may have disregarded. Following a recent change in Department of Defense policy, fourteen states have adopted similar programs.

In Montana, Guard families will be offering the Strong Bronze Program, a three-day marriage retreat with their spouses. "Our chaplain presents ideas about communication, financial stresses, and getting back on the same track with each other," said Wick. "To emphasize the importance we place on it, a soldier can go to this with his spouse in place of a weekend drill."

Hunter said it's important for returning combat vets to be able to talk together, but also to involve their respective families. "In my opinion, the families have been the silent heroes," she said. "They lost a family member to an effort like the Iraq deployment and went through a huge change. As a part of the bigger picture, they also need to be part of the solution to be a support system for the returning Guard member."

Mosley said the retreats will be optional at the 30-, 60-, and 90-day benchmarks after a unit returns from a deployment. Returning soldiers have traditionally been given 90 days off after deployment to spend with their families, but the Montana National Guard has been finding the soldiers need each other during that period as a continuing support group. "But we also found that they didn't need to practice being better soldiers," Mosley said. "They needed to learn how to reintegrate with their families."

Over the past year, the Montana National Guard has adopted the slogan that "Behind every happy soldier is a happy family." "Their efforts have been very impressive," said Hunter. For two days recently, the 120th Fighter Wing's family support group took its place on the processing line as nearly 200 members of the Montana Air National Guard returned from deployment at Balad Air Force Base in Iraq.

"We give family briefings for outgoing and incoming soldiers and their families," said Wick. "We provide a lot of volunteer training, telling them how to be involved here and how to stay in touch with their family member."

The Air National Guard is also handing out a new brochure on post-traumatic stress disorder so soldiers and their families can begin to recognize the symptoms of the emotional disorders caused by combat. That brochure has already gone out to 1,300 to 1,500 Air National Guard families. "Then the Army used it, listed its own local, state, and national resources for PTSD and sent it out to all the Army National Guard families around the state," said Wick. Furthermore, the Air National Guard is distributing a 24-page resource guide on where soldiers can get help for problems they face on their return. It has also gone out to Air and Army National Guard families.

The Montana National Guard has had family readiness units in place in Helena, Great Falls, Missoula, and Glasgow, but has also added units in Kalispell and Belgrade in the past year. "Our family programs are not just available to the National Guard, but to any member of the service having family problems," said Wick.

Some other changes

Today, all less-than-honorable discharges are investigated to make sure they aren't related to combat stress, and Mosley signs off on each one personally if he is convinced it's deserved. Additional suicide prevention and PTSD/mTBI training has been made available throughout the Guard, said Col. Ireland.

All Montana National Guardsmen have been signed up with the VA to allow seamless continuity of care when they retire or leave the service, said Joe Underkofler, director of the state VA Health Care System in Fort Harrison.

Guardsmen have been notified that they can request an honorable discharge due to deployment-related PTSD or mTBI. "We've had some people who said they've been receiving mental health care treatment and don't feel comfortable deploying again, but only a handful of them," said Karlin. Three Montana National Guard units with about 200 soldiers have been put on notice that they may be deployed for a second time within the next year.

"One thing that's clear to me is that the National Guard gets this from the general on down and from the rank and file right back up to the top again," said Matt Kuntz. "The task force came up with a really solid plan, and it's blown me away how well the Guard has taken that plan and put it into action — and in so short a timeframe."

More than one suicide

Shortly after the first anniversary of Chris Dana's suicide, attorneys for the two veterans' groups were arguing in a federal courtroom in California that the VA was deliberately downplaying the number of suicides among military vets. They cited a 2008 *CBS News* report contending that in 2005 alone, there were more than 6,200 suicides among former military personnel. Then they cited the response of Dr. Ira Katz, head of the VA's mental health unit, who challenged the report, saying: "Their number is not, in fact, an accurate reflection of the rate." Finally, the attorneys introduced an email that Katz had written two months before in which he said, "Our suicide prevention coordinators are identifying about 1,000 suicide attempts per month among veterans we see in our medical facilities." And Katz also wrote in the email that the VA is seeing about 18 suicides a day among its 25 million veterans — which is about 6,570 a year. That's also six times higher than the VA had reported just a year earlier.

"I think we ought to be worried," said Senator Patty Murray, D-Washington, noting that only half of the vets with problems have sought treatment and only half of them have received even minimal treatment. "They could be walking time bombs for decades. I hope the VA understands this."

As it turns out, those new VA suicide statistics are about what Jerry Reed, executive director of Washington, DC's Suicide Prevention Action Network (SPAN-USA) would have predicted. He originally was stunned by the fact that one in five suicides in the state of Virginia involved veterans; then he began finding that death rates from other states bore out that prevalence rate.

"It was not necessarily vets from the current era who were committing suicide," he told me. "It was the older vets, the Vietnam-era vets, and I began to wonder if this was a result of living with trauma for so many years. I began to look for that data and found it was replicated in many other states."

America has 32,000 suicides a year, more deaths annually than caused by either AIDS or homicides. Twenty percent of that would be the 6,700 vets that Dr. Kaplan spoke about. Ironically, we have more vets killing themselves each year than we have soldiers actually dying in combat.

Reed also noted that the warning signs for suicide — a feeling of hopelessness, being trapped with no way out, plus an increasing isolation from family and friends — closely mirror those of PTSD.

In addition to an alcoholism rate 50 percent above the national average, Montana also has one of the highest rates of suicide for older white males. Montana, Nevada, Wyoming, and Idaho lead the nation in that category, Reed said. While Reed looked at factors like people per square mile and divorce rates that isolate people, I think it's no coincidence that Montana also has one of the nation's highest ratios of veterans per capita.

"It takes a community to prevent suicide, and Montana has clearly taken a lead there. The National Guard deserves a tremendous amount of credit for taking that lead," Reed said. "You have a success story in Montana. It's true that a huge ship doesn't turn around quickly, but perhaps it turns more quickly in a small community like Montana."

Expanding the outreach

Nearly 16 months after Dana's suicide, Montana's National Guard expanded its PTSD outreach efforts, hosting a series of 20 public meeting in armories across the state. As part of its effort to familiarize the public — and veterans in particular — with post-traumatic stress disorder, it played a video produced at Fort Harrison entitled "Picking Up the Pieces." That had Tiffany Kolar wiping her eyes. "It raised a lot of questions for me," Kolar said after one of the first meetings. "I have a brother who served with the Idaho National Guard and who later committed suicide. Now I'm learning a lot about what must have been happening."

Kolar's husband is currently serving his second tour of duty in Iraq, and she and her mother-in-law need to understand the danger signs, she said. "There were some things we didn't recognize the last time he came home so we want to be better informed this time," said Darlene Kolar, his mother.

Only a handful of people showed up for the meeting here, but the Guard's personnel officer, Col. Ireland, said he was happy for any attention. "If these meetings are able to help even one person, for all the time and effort we've expended, it's been worth it," Ireland said. The Guard sent out personal invitations and videos to 2,000 behavioral health care specialists in Montana, as well as to all the veterans' organizations. Next on the list is a mass mailing to all ministers and religious leaders in the state.

As a direct result of Dana's suicide, Montana is now providing longer mental health assessments after return from combat, strengthening its family support units, creating crisis readiness teams to investigate abnormal behavior, requiring a personal investigation by the adjutant general before any soldier is discharged less than honorably, and producing and promoting its own video. "The Montana National Guard is leading the nation in this regard," said Ireland. "We're doing things that no other state is doing, and we're considered a national model."

The powerful video features two soldiers talking about their emotional problems, with a counselor discussing danger signs. There's also an admission by Dana's stepbrother Kuntz that he let the floundering soldier down by not intervening more strongly to get him help. "We needed a powerful video to be able to reach out and tell our soldiers that we're trying to help them, not punish them for coming home from combat with an [emotional] wound," Ireland said.

Major John Allen, a chaplain who serves as minister of Redeemer Lutheran Church in Great Falls, reinforced the same message. "We wanted to educate people about PTSD and destigmatize it so people can seek help instead of avoiding it," said Allen. For that reason, the public meetings are open to all vets, not just former members of the National Guard; the family readiness units will help families from any branch of the service.

After the formal presentation, Mike Waite of Montana Congressman Denny Rehberg's staff asked about the danger signs of PTSD, including a vet's need to live dangerously and have a weapon within reach. "Soldiers who admitted to PTSD after Vietnam couldn't be promoted, so none of them ever admitted to it," said John Foster, a retired counselor. "I hope all that has changed."

"Yes, it has changed," responded Ireland. "But the military culture changes slowly, so it's important to keep pushing that change." And Michael Stuehm said he currently treats about 30 vets with PTSD at the South Central Montana Regional Mental Health Center in Lewistown. Any additional resources available to him are welcome, he said. "It's great that the National Guard is reaching out to these vets," said Stuehm. "When I came back from Vietnam, there was nothing, so we've come a long way."

I have to agree — discussing and treating PTSD within the Montana National Guard is a remarkable (and oh, so logical) improvement. Without help, this can be a crippling disorder, so caring for your troops requires that you treat the wounds, both physical and emotional. Montana is taking a lead that needs to be followed.

But when you think about it, that's simply good business sense. It's a way of protecting an asset, much the same as a pesticide protects a lovely lawn. What strikes me as most remarkable is that the Guard has taken its concern outside the ranks of active-duty soldiers and into the community as a whole. By telling the vets and their families that there's help for their long-term problems, this effort goes beyond just good business sense and into a genuinely good practice. For thousands of suffering vets, it opens the doors to help.

- 17 -
Conventional treatment

Conventional treatment is, well, conventional. It includes things like individual counseling, group therapy, and lots of medications. The question is whether we should limit ourselves to providing conventional treatment in unconventional times.

For PTSD victims, treatment is critical to improvement. Without treatment within a year or two of a traumatic event, the prognosis for people who continue to experience symptoms is considered to be quite poor. Most conventional modes of treatment, including those used by the VA, involve a combination of group therapies, cognitive behavioral therapies, and/or medicines to realign the chemistry of the brain.

It's also becoming clear that having social support systems in place for a returning combat vet can be a significant factor in his or her ultimate readjustment into society. Often, that involves talking with other vets about their experiences. As group members begin to share a trust with each other, they can share their feelings and discuss how they cope with trauma-related shame, guilt, rage, fear, doubt, and self-condemnation. Sharing those fears allows vets to know they're not alone; sharing the coping strategies gives them ways to deal with painful situations. Throughout the nation, the VA offers a number of vets' listening sessions in which they share experiences, concerns, worries, and a lot of advice. Families, friends, churches, and sports teams can also be invaluable, although soldiers share a special bond with their war buddies. Social support appears to be so helpful that researchers believe it can alleviate some of the genetic predispositions to depression and PTSD.

Cognitive behavioral therapy operates on the theory that trauma is secondary to the perception of trauma. In other words, we all perceive situations differently, and we act on those perceptions. If we can change the way we perceive past threats, we can change the way we deal with them in the present. These include therapies called prolonged exposure, cognitive processing, and stress inoculation. Each helps a vet recover from past traumas.

Cognitive behavioral therapy, which has been around for half a century or more, involves thinking about the way you act and trying to lessen learned responses to certain situations. If, for example, you hit the ground at the sight and sound of a helicopter, you may want to question the value of that behavior in civilian life to remove your fears. By removing the thinking patterns that are wrong in a civilian world, the theory is that we can also change our behavior.

Exposure therapy is one form of cognitive behavioral therapy. Therapists question PTSD victims at length about their traumas in a safe setting to help them face and gain control over the fear and anxiety that initially overwhelmed them. Frequently, they'll take the trauma piece by piece, desensitizing the victim as they work up to the most stressful portions. It's like going through a car wreck again and again and again, and many vets want no part of that ongoing pain. The opposite approach to desensitization is called flooding — it involves bringing out a lot of bad memories all at once, and it teaches people not to feel overwhelmed.

Virtual reality is an exposure therapy that's been around for a decade or more, but it's becoming more sophisticated. One study found that

Vietnam vets' symptoms were reduced by 34 percent when they were treated with a "Virtual Vietnam" program developed at Georgia Tech. A study of rats about five years ago showed that a drug called D-cycloserine (DCS) helped them deal with fear, apparently by calming down the amygdala. In 2004, researchers at Emory University in Atlanta found the drug worked with people, too. People afraid of heights took the drug, then donned virtual reality goggles that shot them skyward in a virtual glass elevator; they found their fear of heights was diminished for up to three months. Dr. Barbara Rothbaum, head of Emory's Trauma and Anxiety Recovery Program, told the Atlanta *Journal-Constitution* that she thinks the drug will also work with vets. "It's just too cool," she said. "It makes the therapy work better and faster. And we're going to need better therapy because these wars are going to cause so much PTSD it's unimaginable. We've just got to find a better and faster way to treat these symptoms."

Now Emory is using a Virtual Iraq model in which returning vets don a VR helmet to see themselves behind the wheel or in the passenger seat of a Humvee. They hear explosions, or they see insurgents popping up and firing AK-47s at them. Grenades whiz in as planes or helicopters fly over. Smoke pillars rise. And a Nintendo joystick lets them steer their way through the perils, but not fire back. Aaron Beach, a 23-year-old Iraqi vet in treatment at Emory, told the newspaper: "It puts you back there for sure. The stuff doesn't look totally real, but it all feels real. It's scary. You sweat like an E-5 trying to read!"

Along with the exposure therapy, cognitive restructuring involves identifying and getting rid of negative thoughts. There are some learned skills for coping with anxiety, such as focusing on breathing. There are techniques for managing anger, including timeouts and safe places. Stress inoculation is a way of anticipating upcoming problems and preparing to deal with them safely. And rebuilding communication skills is imperative, particularly when a marriage is at risk.

Meds can restore proper chemical balance

Pharmaceuticals are also a part of the conventional treatment, and many vets have a small arsenal of pills to control different mood swings. One local Vietnam vet gave me a list of eight different medications that he takes every day — some for pain, some for anxiety, and some antidepressants. One problem is that medications may do one thing when taken alone, but operate differently in combination with other drugs.

The *American Journal of Psychiatry* lists about two dozen pharmaceuticals that can be used to alleviate PTSD symptoms. There are five selective serotonin reuptake inhibitors (SSRIs) that have been shown to be effective in reducing intrusive recollections, avoidance/numbing, and hyperarousal; side effects can include insomnia, restlessness, nausea, sexual dysfunction, and nervousness or anxiety. Four other secondary antidepressants may do almost as well with fewer side effects. Phenelzine can reduce intrusive recollections, depression, panic disorder, and social phobia, although patients are required to follow a strict diet to avoid hypertension. It doesn't work in combination with other antidepressants, central nervous system stimulants, decongestants, or alcohol. Three tricyclic antidepressants can help reduce nightmares and flashbacks, while four other antiadrenergic drugs can reduce intrusive recollections and hyperarousal. Five anticonvulsants may do the same, with different side effects, and three atypical antipsychotic drugs may be effective against a cluster of PTSD symptoms and aggression.

Selective serotonin reuptake inhibitors are among the most popular medications for PTSD treatment because they have been shown to significantly reduce the symptoms. Conversely, discontinuation of the treatments has been associated with clinical relapse and a return of the original symptoms. One SSRI, paroxetine, may have promise in reducing cognitive defects among PTSD victims. Researchers tested memory and hippocampus volume among patients who had used paroxetine for nine to 12 months and found both significant improvement in logical, figural, and visual memory, and also a 4.6 percent increase in the volume of the hippocampus. However, there's still a lot of room for improvement — only 30 percent of the patients using SSRIs achieved full remission of symptoms.

Researchers are also experimenting with a new drug that apparently blocks memories — or at least blocks out the worst of them. James McGaugh, a professor of neurobiology in Irvine, Texas, began experimenting with propranolol after he observed that lab rats charged up with adrenaline remembered things better than rats without that adrenaline high. Propranolol blocks some of that adrenaline, so he designed an experiment involving rats swimming randomly in a tank of water that had a clear plastic surface just below the water line. When they found it, they climbed aboard immediately. And the next day, they went looking for it and found it a little faster. Then McGaugh administered a shot of adrenaline to a rat that had just found the platform, and the next day, the rat swam to it immediately. So the next time, he administered a shot of propranolol, and the rat swam around the tank without any indication it remembered finding the surface the previous day. "Propranolol sits on that nerve cell and blocks it, so that, think of this being a key and this being a lock; the hole in the lock is blocked because of the propranolol sitting there," McGaugh told *CBS News*. "So adrenaline can be present, but it can't do its job."

At Harvard, Roger Pitman read McGaugh's rat studies and immediately thought of its application for PTSD. "When I read this, I said, 'This has got to be how post-traumatic stress disorder operates,' because think about what happens to a person," he told CBS. "First of all, they have a horribly traumatic event, and they have intense fear and helplessness. So that intense fear and helplessness is gonna stimulate adrenaline. And then what do we find three months or six months or 20 years later? Excessively strong memories." So Pitman began experimenting with human beings who had recently been traumatized, trying to administer propranolol as soon as possible after the trauma had occurred. That work got Pitman funded for a larger study by the National Institutes of Health, although the President's Council on Bioethics raised a concern that rewriting memories with drugs may undermine the victim's true identity.

But researchers emphasize that the drug will only lower the intensity of a bad memory — not erase it. "It's not that people will no longer remember the trauma, but the memory will be less painful," Alain Brunet, a psychologist at McGill University, told the Chicago *Tribune*. At McGill, Karim Nader, a pioneering psychologist, began to find that memories are changeable each time they're used. "It was formerly thought that once a memory is fixed, you can't mess around with it. That was scientific dogma for 100 years," he told the *Tribune*. Instead, he found that emotional memories are more intense because they cause stress-related hormones like adrenaline to be released by the amygdala. He speculated that PTSD may be a result of the trauma overwhelming the amygdala and creating memories with too high a level of emotional gain. Propranolol blocks some of that emotional charge and allows the person to remember those traumatic events like a bystander, not a participant. McGaugh told the *Tribune*, "Many people have thought of these as amnesia drugs: 'I would like to get rid of the memory of a horrible experience I had with another person; I'll just take propranolol and get rid of it.' Well, propranolol does not get rid of memories." He recalled getting a phone call from a woman who wanted to know if she could erase the memory of her abusive first husband. "The idea of erasing a memory is just silly," Nader told the *Tribune*. "We can't do it, nor do we want to. But if we can turn down the intensity of the memory sufficiently that these people can respond to traditional treatments, that's the goal."

But there's also a widespread concern that pharmaceuticals may be used to mask deficiencies in the way these disorders are diagnosed and treated. "In general, the most effective regimen of treatment for psychological wounds is one-on-one therapy, combined with other treatment means such as medication and group therapy," said Bobby Muller, president of Veterans for America. "Given the dearth of mental health care providers, service members with combat-related mental wounds are often primarily treated through medication rather than primarily through one-on-one care from the same mental health care provider."

That has to change, said Muller. "We are facing a massive mental health problem as a result of our wars in Iraq and Afghanistan. As a country, we have not responded adequately to this problem. Unless we act urgently and wisely, we'll be dealing with an epidemic of service-connected psychological wounds for years to come."

Need to move forward

But Dr. Peake, the head of the VA, is an advocate of conservative medicine. "Exposure therapy and cognitive behavioral therapy are the practices being promulgated," he told me. "What we really want to do is keep moving forward toward evidence-based medicine." While there are some different therapies that claim success in treating PTSD, they make the doctor nervous. "I don't know that they have any research protocols," he said. "We need to look very hard at the control studies and scientific evidence. We have a responsibility to our vets to make sure that what we do and what we provide has a quality basis to it."

- 18 -
Healing through faith

Turning to religion to ask for forgiveness also seems to help. Faces of Combat turn to the face of God as the beginning of the search for a new meaning in life.

Hardie Higgins doesn't believe in medications. "Pharmaceuticals are just a mask because they don't deal with a problem. They just cover it up. You can get the same thing with alcohol and drugs. I just don't think that helps," he told me, "but then I'm not a doctor."

Higgins is a retired Army lieutenant colonel, with 20 years as a chaplain under his belt. He has written his Ph.D. thesis on PTSD and knows his subject first-hand, having served tours of duty in both Vietnam and Iraq. In fact, he had begun to realize some of the effects of mild PTSD after his own return from 'Nam, experiencing one of those magical moments in which you're transported from one life to another with no time for decompression. "I'd flown out of Camron Bay to Fort

Lewis to Denver," he said. "As I was taking a shower that night, cleaning the dirt and dust of Vietnam off me, I remember watching that dirt go down the drain and thinking, 'There goes a year of my life down the drain.' Then as I was eating breakfast the next morning, I realized I had absolutely no emotion. I was watching a school bus go by and thought to myself that if that bus catches on fire with all those kids on it, the only emotion I'll feel is whether I can get some catsup for my potatoes."

In his unpublished doctoral thesis, Higgins writes about the aftermath of 'Nam. "Though I was in a deep sleep, I could hear the distant sound of rockets hitting the air base at Da Nang about four miles away. In my half-awake stupor, I thought to myself they would surely sound the alarm and require us to get out of our bunks and go for the bunkers. The air base received hits three or four times a week, but that was as close to us as the rockets ever got. Every time they fired at the base, we had to get up, put our clothes on, and head to the bunker for about an hour. What a waste of sleeping time. The immediate, loud WHAAP-WHAAP of two 122mm rockets exploding about 200 meters to the south engaged my trained instincts. I rapidly rolled off the top bunk and pulled Mike Dilts off and covered him with my body.

"Then I heard a feminine voice softly speak, 'Wow.' I was sitting upright and I glanced to my left to see my wife lying in our bed in Kansas. It was 2 a.m. and the plastic front grill of the air conditioner I had purchased two days earlier had fallen off and hit the wooden floor with a loud WHAAP. My wife described my 'levitating straight up about a foot, arms straight out to my side, then sitting bolt upright, eyes wide open and staring off in some distant place.'"

Higgins is convinced that recovery lies in a combination of Christian faith and finding meaning in both the suffering you've been through and in the rest of your life.

In many ways, Vietnam and Iraq were a lot alike. "The stress wasn't necessarily in being a combat soldier," he says. "Just being in the arena of combat is stress enough because you never know what's going to come at you. The other stress is the poverty of a third-world country. It's a total cultural change. During five months in Iraq, I saw a lot of the same things I saw in Vietnam. One difference is that a lot of the Vietnam kids had a stronger faith-based belief in right or wrong. Today's generation is more individual morality. But trauma is still about a loss of meaning, who they are, what they're about, and their purpose in life."

Another loss is the familiar lifestyle that soldiers had been accustomed to at home. Just being in Vietnam or Iraq has a nightmarish quality to it, a surreal feeling. "The jungles of Vietnam had their oppressive heat and humidity combined with layers of canopy to prevent much light or the slightest breeze to penetrate the floor. The rice paddies were usually filled with water and fertilized with human and animal excrement and bred countless biting insects and leeches. Most soldiers, upon arriving at an airfield and stepping off the plane commented almost immediately about the stench that attacked their nostrils," writes Higgins. "In the Middle East, the searing heat and desert sand combined with third-world living conditions give the soldier a true sense of 'This isn't Kansas, Toto.' With a daily heat index ranging from 125 to 140 degrees in the middle of the summer and the very cold nights of January and February combined with the weekly sandstorms that creep into every crevice and item of equipment, comfort is a relative perception. In the middle of summer on patrol, a soldier drinks only hot water from a plastic bottle. Water is hot enough that she or he can add instant coffee to it and have a cup with no problem. The soldiers work 14- to 16-hour shifts with constant threat of mortar attacks to the living compounds and of improvised explosive devices on the roadways. Insects and diseases indigenous to the region add to the discomfort for many soldiers."

And in this unreal atmosphere, combat destroys the moral rules soldiers grew up with. "They lose their 'Thou shalt not kill' to what becomes an adrenaline high," Higgins added. For some of them, it becomes an addictive high. They know what the rules are on the battlefield, but when they come back, it's much harder. That's why the re-enlistment rates in-theater are so astronomical. They've lost their meaning at home, and the only meaning they have left is with their combat buddies."

Higgins calls it psychic numbing. "They become so numb they lose all emotion," he said. "The only emotion they can feel is in a combat zone with the bonding of their buddies. It's almost like the drug addict having to have the ultimate high to stay normal. When they get home, their environment is so uneventful that these young soldiers have to drive their cars at 100 mph, drink to insensibility, and push themselves to the limit. Consequently, the amount of self-inflicted injuries is, if not astronomical, at least very significant."

Guilt is a huge part of the problem, he believes. Wartime bonding is critical, and losing a buddy means that you didn't watch his back well enough. Young soldiers going into combat talk about their fear, but it's less about being killed or being wounded than it is of letting their buddies down at a critical time by being unable to do what they need to do. "Sometimes young soldiers go berserk under combat and begin ravaging with their weapons — whatever moves is dead because my buddy is dead." And there are the normal consequences of war to deal with. "When you take a house out, you may find you've taken a man out, but there are four children left crippled by your gunfire. There's a moral conundrum in combat. Soldiers are there knowing what they're trained to do, hoping they won't have to do it, but doing it anyway."

So with the physical destruction comes a destruction of meaning. Many soldiers come out of combat with a feeling that there is no real purpose or possibility of measurable progress. Patrolling the same ground over and over again for no reason leads to that feeling. So does torching poverty-stricken villages or blowing up abandoned homes just for the sake of doing something. "Within this anti-meaning is a profound loss of personal dignity that is stripped from the soldier by the horror, waste, and trauma experienced in combat," Higgins writes. "Whether the soldier is the recipient of the horror, waste, and trauma through observation, loss of a friend, personal wounds, or a perpetrator through acts of violence or rage, the soldier recognizes there is no dignity around, through, or to him. Without dignity, there can be no assurance that life is worth living."

And with that loss comes a destruction of morality. "That which disturbs the veteran suffering from PTSD is not so much what happened in his or her past as it is what Viktor Frankl calls the 'existential vacuum' created by the event over and against the belief system that the soldier held prior to the event," said Higgins. That makes a soldier feel totally alone. There's a mild paranoia in which the soldier begins to fear that his leaders and his buddies will begin to see the emptiness within him and perceive it to be a weakness. And he begins to perceive it as a weakness, as well.

One solution is forgiveness

To help soldiers lift their burden of guilt, the chaplain turns to the Bible, to a forgiving God who requires that we also forgive others and forgive ourselves as He forgives us. As the Lord's Prayer says, "Forgive us our trespasses, as we forgive those who trespass against us." But that's nowhere near as easy as it sounds. Higgins sometimes sits soldiers down in a chair and asks them to talk to the people they've wronged, then asks them to take the opposite chair to be the victim addressing the soldier.

When a soldier believes that God will forgive him, others will forgive him, and he can forgive himself, then comes a search for new meaning in his life. That requires a vet to find some meaning for the suffering he experienced in war and to find a way to use that suffering in a civilian world. "The key to recovery for victims of PTSD is, I believe, to assist them in discovering the redemptive meaning of their suffering and how to use that suffering to add meaning to their future life," Higgins said.

"Assisting them in discovering the future meaning in their lives by addressing their psychic numbing or nihilism, anti-meaning, desensitization, or existential vacuum is the focus of the treatment through Logotherapy toward initiating recovery for the soldier. The program, though ontologically driven by the traumatic event, focuses on the teleological restoration of meaning or purpose in the victim's life. Dwelling upon the event through repeated re-telling of the story can provide a catharsis in some cases; however, it also reinforces the victimization of the individual in many cases. Therefore, turning the focus away from the event and toward the desired outcome does not negate the event — rather it reinforces the recovery."

Logotherapy is a treatment first advocated by Frankl, a survivor of four Nazi prison camps (including Auschwitz in Poland), that uses a soldier's own religious metaphors to open and clean out the festering memories so he can grow spiritually, said Higgins. It requires a solid theology of the sovereignty of God and an understanding that suffering is necessary in all of our lives. While God permits evil, it's only so that people have a choice to turn to good … and the choice to turn to God.

The first step in Logotherapy is self-distancing, which requires a vet to begin thinking of his previous combat as an observer, rather than a participant. Focusing on the problem only causes the patient to identify more and more with the symptoms, Higgins believes, so it's important to transcend the past and focus on the future. The second is to change his attitudes. One important change for a vet is to realize he or she has survived. That moves the individual from a victim to a victor, from being traumatized to being triumphant. With that should come a reduction in PTSD symptoms.

But the real cure is to find a meaning in life for what he has been through, a meaning that defines life beyond the suffering experience itself. Frequently, that requires developing a sense of mission or meaning in life. It also requires them to stop focusing on themselves and to begin being of service to others. That's also a Biblical admonition: "Love thy neighbor as thyself."

Socratic questioning can be useful, but so can another technique that Frankl introduced called the paradoxical intention, which is basically the antithesis of the self-fulfilling prophesy. When a patient has a claustrophobic fear of elevators and fears he would faint in one, the counselor encourages him to take an elevator and try to faint. When he finds he can't, he's free of that fear. He has disarmed the anticipatory anxiety that feeds the neurosis.

Deep-seated guilt comes out in nightmares

One of the vets Higgins has counseled recently is Melvin Osburn, who saw a lot of action in Vietnam but locked it away in his mind. "I've made a lot of choices, and I've paid the consequences for them for years and years," said Osburn. "I was driving down the road outside of our camp with another supply sergeant, a guy who was kind of like a young punk. A sniper shot out our windshield, and this guy fell into my lap. I thought he was dead. I couldn't slow down or speed up. All of a sudden, he sat up and said, 'Get the hell out of here.' It was months before I could get that windshield replaced because it was the monsoon season over there.

The first day I got that new windshield, I was driving down the same road and a sniper shot it out again. I was so mad I stopped in the middle of the road and chased that sniper down. When I caught him, I realized that I'd left my own weapon in the jeep, so I beat his brains out with his own weapon."

But two incidents came back to haunt Osburn, incidents that he never told anyone about because he feared being court-martialed.

The first incident involved missing laundry. A supply truck took dirty laundry to be washed, but there were sheets and pillowcases that were missing afterward. Suspecting that kids were stealing them, Osburn said he hid in the back of the truck with his rifle to see what was going on. "One of the supply sergeants said just knock them off the truck if they get in it. I didn't want to hurt anyone, but I heard a bunch of kids outside the truck. Then they threw this little kid into the truck, and I hit him with the butt of my rifle and splattered his brains out." Killing a civilian, particularly a little kid, was a potentially serious problem, so Osburn kept his mouth shut about it for years.

The second issue was that he accidentally shot a fellow soldier and may have killed him. In Saigon, he became friends with one Sgt. Wilson, a Special Forces soldier who said he was taking a patrol out one night. He invited Osburn to join them, and Osburn did, even though he had no permission. "In fact, I was AWOL," he said. "We got ambushed that night, and I was standing on the chest of one of those guys and stabbing him with my bayonet when I heard a noise behind me and whirled around and shot Sgt. Wilson. I helped load him into the helicopter and got in with him and held him in my arms. I was crying and saying that by God, I'd never get close to anyone again in my life. When the helicopter landed, I jumped out, ran to my Jeep, and went back to camp. I could have been court-martialed over that one, too, so I never told anyone about it."

Memories and nightmares tormented him for years, Osburn said. In the mid-1980s, he woke up crying and couldn't stop. His wife found him in tears in the living room, and he finally was able to confess what he'd done. A decade later, he began dreaming that one of his own grandkids was the little boy he killed with the butt of his rifle. His pastor recommended PTSD treatment, so Osburn spent six weeks in treatment in Oklahoma City. "The psychiatrist suggested I put in a claim with the government, but they denied it because they had no proof of all the things I'd done," he said.

Recently, Higgins began counseling him. "He sat me down and asked me to pretend that Sgt. Wilson was in the chair opposite mine," said Osburn. "I started crying and asked him to forgive me just like I would have if he'd actually been sitting there. Then he had me switch chairs and be Sgt. Wilson, and I heard him telling me that he forgave me. One of the last things he told me before we went out on patrol was, 'Okie, no matter what happens out there tonight, don't ever walk away from God.' Then as we were sitting in the chairs, he said 'I heard you swear to God you'd never let anyone get close to you again, and that really hurt me.' Hearing Sgt. Wilson forgive me helped me more than the whole six weeks of treatment I received in Oklahoma City."

Higgins did the same thing with Osburn talking to the little boy. "He explained to the kid that he was just a soldier doing his job and he was sorry. Then I put him in the other chair and said, 'Now you're the little kid. What do you want to say to the soldier?' And it was amazing how much more forgiving the kid was. He said, 'I know you were just a soldier and you didn't know what you were doing.' When you hear that kid talking about forgiveness, there's some real healing going on."

That moral conundrum

Combat violates the morality that the soldiers grew up with, so I had to wonder why Higgins had remained in the Army for four decades. When I asked him, his answer was two-fold. First, he said because that's where he was needed most. And second, it's where the worst problems were. Furthermore, Christian values should be everywhere, including the military. "Would you want a soldier who didn't hold Christian values, who didn't have a firm sense of what is right?" he asks. "Just because you're a soldier, you shouldn't have to forfeit your Christian beliefs. Would you want mercenaries protecting our country?"

Unfortunately, mercenaries *are* protecting our country. The so-called private security contractors are ex-service members working for private companies and making a lot of money out of war, which is the definition of a mercenary. And I think my question remains a valid one. Most of us would feel justified in killing someone who is attempting to kill us, so I suspect there was less of a moral conflict in defending America against invasion and aggression during World Wars I and II. But Vietnam raised a lot of issues for me because I felt America was the aggressor, invading someone else's country. My response to that was to accept being drafted in 1968, but to search for a place in the Army where I wouldn't be required to participate in a combat that I had grave doubts about — I guess I was simply begging the question: if it was wrong for *me*, how could I abet a system that required others to unjustly kill or be killed? I feel the same way about the current war. I believe the Bush administration lied to the American people to suck us into what's essentially Vietnam II. Sadly, much of the rest of the world also condemns our actions in Iraq and Afghanistan. I suspect that makes it harder for our soldiers because it increases their moral qualms about what they're being required to do.

- 19 -
Helping the brain adjust

Neurotherapy helps reduce the symptoms of PTSD. The VA is not currently allowing the treatment to be used in some government facilities. However, private practitioners are using it with success and hope to convince the VA to change its current position.

As has been mentioned, there are some very interesting treatment options, but not all of them are available to combat vets through the VA, a government agency that can be cautious, stodgy, and bureaucratic. One of them is a new form of neurotherapy, Alpha-Stim, now offered through the Rimrock Foundation of Billings, Montana. Rimrock has been offering neurotherapy to civilians for the past few years after it lost its government contract to provide care to combat vets. Rimrock treated 176 combat vets between 2002 and 2004 before the VA switched its contract to Billings Mental Health. "If we'd had Alpha-Stim [direct electrical stimulation of the brain] when we were doing our vets, every one of them would have been on this," Mona Sumner, Rimrock's chief operations officer, told me.

Rimrock is finding that this therapy is working wonders with abused women suffering from PTSD, as well as drug addicts and alcoholics. It said neurotherapy cuts down on the desire to use drugs, as well as reducing stress, anxiety, depression, and insomnia.

In a short session, that relief came to Mandy Smith, who suffers from post-traumatic stress disorder and seeks help from the thoughts shooting uncontrollably through her mind. It's been a day of tears and anger for this 24-year-old abuse victim and former drug addict, who can feel the tension in her forehead and all but see the etched lines that arch up across her forehead from the bridge of her nose.

Soft music is playing and the lights are dim as Smith plugs onto each earlobe an electrode attached to a device resembling an iPod. Her session will be 20 minutes.

Developed by Dr. Daniel L. Kirsch, onetime clinical director of the Center for Pain and Stress-Related Disorders at Columbia-Presbyterian Hospital in New York City, the device blows a gentle electrical current through her brain. It has the same frequency as an alpha brainwave, the state that people who meditate seek to achieve. It's described as being awake but relaxed, the peace you feel on awakening or just before going to sleep.

The current is believed to stimulate groups of nerve cells located near the stem of the brain. Those clusters produce neurotransmitters (serotonin and acetylcholine), which modulate brain activity.

"This has been a brutal week for me because of a relationship I was in and because I'm having delusional thoughts of an eating disorder," said Smith as the treatment begins. "Now that I don't drink or do drugs anymore, the eating disorder is a way of messing up my head."

After her best friend died in a car wreck at 15, Smith became an alcoholic and then a drug addict. Now she's in recovery. "I've been smoking a lot of cigarettes this week, and I've been isolating because I don't want to be around people," she said.

Therapist Shelly Hocking sits with Smith, watching her face for signs of relaxation. "For the first three or four minutes, my thoughts were just racing," Smith said. "But now I'm feeling some relief."

One intrusive thought is often the brutal beating she took outside a Phoenix, Arizona, crack house before dawn one morning a few years ago. "It was just a total act of violence," she said. "He beat me nearly to death, stabbed me eight times, including one good shot to the arm that went in one side and out the other."

By now, the treatment is beginning to work. "Before this started, I was thinking about a lot of things, but now I'm just focusing on this conversation," Smith said.

Although she survived the assault, Smith has seen her share of death as she abused LSD, cocaine, and methamphetamines. "I saw one friend die who was drinking and driving," she said. "He was racing and wrapped his car around a tree. We ran up to pull him out, but he was gargling blood so it was no use."

With about four minutes left in her treatment, the tension lines in Smith's forehead dissolve and she just looks terribly tired. "I've been medicated for years, but this is the best way of dealing with this anxiety," she said. "You feel a lot better, and you're not numb."

For Rimrock's Mona Sumner, the therapy is simply extraordinary. "Mandy is pretty much a miracle child," she said. "Her disease (addiction) is so far progressed that our staff says she doesn't have one more relapse in her. If she relapses again, she'll be dead."

Lasting benefits

After the session, the peace can remain for days. Patients who have been stabilized usually use the machine once or twice a week, Sumner said. "This particular intervention has been one of the most significant therapies that we've found. It was a defining moment for the Rimrock Foundation when we began to use it."

It's particularly helpful for treating depression, anxiety, and insomnia, all of which are symptoms of PTSD, said Jon Gjersing, Rimrock's director of nursing. Also called cranial electrotherapy stimulation, Alpha-Stim has been approved by the U.S. Food and Drug Administration as a treatment. Stimulators cost $400 to $600, and are available only with a doctor's prescription.

The Center for Mental Health in Great Falls, which has one of the VA contracts to treat combat vets, doesn't offer neurotherapy; its medical director, Dr. Michael Mason, said he was unfamiliar with Alpha-Stim. Teresa Bell, spokeswoman for the VA at Fort Harrison, said the agency doesn't normally use neurotherapy as a treatment. Instead, it relies on cognitive therapy, medications, and a program called Vet-to-Vet in which combat vets help each other with common problems.

But Gjersing said it has proven valuable in treating depression. "Statistics show that 65 percent of all people in treatment suffer from depression," he said.

With PTSD, the brain is hyperactive and can't slow itself down, he added. "A lot of people go from the sleep mode directly into the anxiety mode. This machine sets up a low-frequency radio wave, and the brain responds to it by slowing down." The anxiety will probably return in hours or days, but not as severely as it did before, said Gjersing.

It's also effective on traumatic brain injuries, said Sumner, adding, "It seems to target the damaged part of the brain to work on." And it can be used to reduce chronic pain, Gjersing said. "It seems to change how the brain processes pain. We do know that depression and anxiety exacerbate pain."

A study group of 3,200 patients in Texas showed no adverse side effects, said Sumner, although it shouldn't be used by patients with medical implants. Rimrock is now using Alpha-Stim on most of the young women it's treating for trauma and drug abuse, Sumner said, "And it's made a tremendous difference for them."

Paranoia becomes bearable

Anxiety attacks have been severe for Cara, a 26-year-old mother of two sons who asked that her last name not be used because she fears her ex-husband, whom she described as a wife-abusing meth dealer. "There's a restraining order against him," she said softly, "but that's only a piece of paper."

At 13, she said, she was molested by an uncle for several years before she ran away and turned to drugs for relief. When she got pregnant, she stopped doing drugs and got married. Meth tore that marriage apart, she said. "I started using meth again shortly before our divorce, but it didn't save our marriage," said Cara.

Actually, it made things worse. He beat her badly, and she had to leave their home in Idaho with their children. "But after I filed for divorce, he wouldn't let it go," Cara said. "He stalked me and the people he sold meth to stalked me. It was a scary time."

Cara came to Montana and sought treatment at Rimrock. She lived in constant terror in a group home with an undisclosed location. "I had to have all the blinds at the house pulled down, and I wouldn't go outside," Cara said. "I had to peek out the windows all the time, keep track of all the cars coming and going, make notes of all the different license plates. Living in a state of fear all the time made my heart race."

The Alpha-Stim treatment has eased that anxiety a lot, she said. "The first two weeks I was here, I couldn't sit and watch a movie with my kids," Cara said. "But now I can sit and relax with them. I know that change is because of the Alpha-Stim because when one of my kids got sick and I missed my treatments for two weeks, I could feel the difference. I was back up at the windows again."

Cara had originally been prescribed Wellbutrin, an antidepressant, but the neurotherapy treatments have been so successful she's quit taking medications. "I'm grateful for that," Cara said. "It numbed me, and I didn't want to be dependant on drugs again."

Shut down by the VA

Keli Remus, who runs Chinook Winds Counseling in Great Falls, is a big fan of Alpha-Stim. "I started using it on September 9," he said. "You know something is working when you can remember the exact day you bought it."

Remus is a counselor who now specializes in PTSD patients under contract to the VA; he started as a sex-abuse counselor. He said that trying to help those victims gave him a secondary case of PTSD. "I was having nightmares four, five, and six times a week," he said. "And nothing helped. But with Alpha-Stim, they're almost gone, down by about 95 percent. I only get one or two a month now."

Based on that personal experience, Remus began using the device on his VA patients and found that it was equally effective. "I was using it on guys who had anxiety and depression. They could calm down and relax so that things registered. Then they began to show a significant change, long-term. I saw that they could think better and function better. One of my guys who struggles with anger was able to remain calm while he sat in a traffic jam."

Unfortunately, when his clients went back down to Fort Harrison for their checkups, they began to talk about how much better they were. "They called me in and ordered me to cease and desist," said Remus. "So I did. Not only will they not pay for this treatment, but they won't even let me use it in any session that the VA pays for. But I'm hoping and praying that the VA will change course and allow me to use it."

Neurofeedback may help normalize the brain

At the EEG Institute in Woodland Hills, California, just north of Los Angeles, counselors use Alpha-Stim to relax patients in the beginning sessions of their treatment, but go far beyond that, clinical director Sue Othner told me. Their treatment is true neurofeedback.

"The essence of neurofeedback is that it's training our brains, fine-tuning them," said Othner. "We're teaching the brain how to shift down to a calmer state and relax."

That involves putting electrodes on a patient and allowing him to play computer games with his emotions. The two calmest brain waves are called alpha and beta, and the patient is working to achieve these calming frequencies. By watching to see what works, the patients learn to control their own brain waves and learn how to quiet their own anxieties.

That's important, Othner said, because the anxiety tends to block the brain from processing the trauma that injured it. "You can replay minor incidents until you defuse them," she said. "But in trauma, it's hard to process anything. The experience sits there unresolved, so it has the weight of an ongoing experience."

Her husband, Siegfried Othner, said PTSD is basically a physiological memory. "The memory of a traumatic event rivets itself into the body-mind, a physiological memory. The whole body recalls the injury. So the remedy lies in restructuring the memory by allowing the person to benignly experience the memory. And that brings about a separation between the body memory and the mind memory. Then the person can go back and visit that memory safely."

The first step is to put the person very much at ease, a state where the body has this healing experience. "We put him in a state just short of sleep. Then the brain ruminates about its own self because the external environment is absent. It ruminates about those traumas. They may come up in a veiled fashion, or they may come up rather vividly. But the brain doesn't go anywhere that a person can't handle because the vivid memories startle the person out of that state," said Siegfried Othner.

The trauma has to come out and be processed before the true healing can take place, Sue Othner said. "In a deep state, you feel safe and calm and relaxed, and your brain can process that trauma. Your brain has wanted to do this work, but it has been blocked by your emotions. So it can be fairly dramatic when those images come forth. I did a session with a Vietnam vet, a medic, who basically saw every bad thing that had happened to him in Vietnam during a 40-minute session. In Vietnam, he was totally devastated, exhausted, covered with sores, and he totally fell apart. After the session, he told me he had developed a totally new image of himself, and that finally allowed him to talk about his experiences."

She said their work builds on the research done during the 1960s by E.G. Peniston, a VA counselor who found neurofeedback very helpful in dealing with Vietnam vets. Now the EEG Institute offers that help free of charge to combat vets with PTSD. "It was clear that it had a huge influence for veterans," said Sue Othner.

But her husband can't figure out why this treatment hasn't been more popular. "We see a couple of veterans at a time, but we should be flooded with them," said Siegfried Othner. "We've got occasional vets, all doing well, but we're not crowded. I don't understand it. It gets to be enormously frustrating."

Unfortunately, the vet that the Othners considered their star patient and recommended for an interview about his success told me he was too stressed out from his dealings with the VA to talk about the treatment.

- 20 -
Reducing the pain

There are some specific treatments, not yet used by the VA, that have helped vets with PTSD. Eye-Movement Desensitization and Reprocessing (EMDR) brings up repressed memories and reprocesses them to cut down on the pain. Emotional Freedom Techniques (EFT) helps veterans reduce or eliminate the pain caused by memories of combat without having to fully relive the event.

Eye-Movement Desensitization and Reprocessing

Eye-Movement Desensitization and Reprocessing (EMDR) has been effective for some vets, although it's primarily a private-practice option that's not available through conventional VA treatment programs.

EMDR is one of the treatments that have been helping Heather Kryszak, who recently ended a nine-year career with the New York National Guard and moved to Chicago. She told me that anxiety, fear, nightmares, depression, and a huge load of anger finally made her realize that she needed help. Normally an outgoing person, she found herself making excuses to avoid her friends, sit at home, and stare mindlessly at a television screen.

And that reminded her of a friend of her dad's back in Holland, New York, a guy who had served two tours of duty in Vietnam and suffered badly from PTSD. "Sometimes we wouldn't see him for a year at a time because he couldn't come out of his house," she said. "He was a prisoner in his own home, and I didn't want to be like that."

For eight or nine months, Kryszak tried to press a claim with the VA, but it was so backlogged that nothing was happening. So she took matters into her own hands and decided to see a private therapist who specialized in EMDR.

"Eye-movement desensitization was really weird," said Kryszak. "I didn't know what to expect, but it brought things out of my memory that I'd been totally suppressing from Iraq. One moment I was laughing and the next moment I was crying."

Kryszak said her therapist would ask how she felt about a certain subject, then ask how strongly she felt about it on a scale of one to ten. Then the therapist would ask her to think about the good feelings or the bad feelings associated with that subject. "Then she'd hold up her hands, move them left or right, and tell me to follow them with my eyes. And then she'd ask me what I was feeling. It was amazing what came out, things from Iraq, things from Bosnia, and things from my childhood."

One of the issues that surfaced was being the only female in a platoon filled with men. "I was never abused — they treated me like a sister," she said. "But I also got a lot of flak that affected my self-esteem. I remember stupid stuff like people telling me that if I didn't pick up their laundry, they wouldn't be my friend any more. And I needed people to be my friends because I had no other friends or family. So some of them took advantage of me."

And there was always an undercurrent of sex, she said. "When you're a girl in the Army, there are only so many of us and most of us don't get along. Girls that join the Army tend to hate other girls, so you have no other choice than to make friends with the guys. But the minute you're spending time with male soldiers, something else is going on and you can't just be friends. That's the hardest part of being in the Army. If you're spending time with a guy, people believe you're really screwing around. I never did any of that, though — I was too busy trying to stay alive.

"But now I realize that some of those people really weren't my friends," said Kryszak. "And as I go through therapy, I'm beginning to realize that it's OK not to like them."

When friends die

Bosnia wasn't too bad for Kryszak. She didn't fear for her life every day as she did in Iraq where she was a military policeman with the National Guard's 105th MP from Buffalo, New York. "Losing two of my friends was the hardest part of Iraq for me," she said. "Both were killed in IED attacks. I knew Heath had a wife and an unborn child. I was on the radio, and we heard the explosions, which weren't that far away. Hearing it all on the radio and being so helpless was the worst. At first, all we had was a KIA [killed in action], no name. When we found out it was Heath, I didn't believe it or want to believe it. We were all in a zombie phase, going through the motions. We held a little ceremony, but after that there was no more time to mourn because we all had to push through."

Next to die was Mike Williams, one of those go-to guys who hold a whole unit together with a positive attitude that's contagious. "Mikie was a great, great guy, friends with everyone," said Kryszak. "When we lost him, the company morale went down to zero. For a good three weeks, no one could function."

Both deaths were senseless and unnecessary, said Kryszak, because the New York National Guard was not properly equipped for battle in Iraq. It had Kevlar helmets and flak jackets, she said, but the Humvees in which both of her friends died lacked armor plating.

"If we'd had the proper equipment, we wouldn't have lost those guys, so there's a lot of anger in me," she said. Then, after a pause to think about it: "Even as I'm sitting here now, my hands are clenched, and

I'm ready to punch someone out because that should not have happened."

That anger, frequently fueled by fear, would grow and grow during Kryszak's tour of duty, as it did the morning she turned on two of her friends for no really good reason, just because she was in a foul mood. "We were escorting fuel trucks from Scania to Baghdad," she said. "We got the trucks all lined up, ready to move out. I was in the lead vehicle with a lieutenant and a gunner. We waited until all the trucks moved out of camp, then gunned it to get up to the front so we could be the scout vehicle. Just as we were about to pass the lead vehicle, an IED went off, a big black cloud of smoke that hit the truck. It had been buried on the side of the road between two palm trees, and it put a huge hole in the ground. The whole windshield of the truck was totally spider glass, the side window was shattered, and there were holes here and there. The trucks were still able to roll, so we just turned around and headed back to base camp."

But fear and guilt were overwhelming, said Kryszak. "It had hit a truck that had two of my really good friends in it, but it could have been me in that truck if they'd been a second slower or we'd been a second faster. I'd been really mean to both of them that day, and when we got back to base camp, I jumped out of the truck crying and said, 'I'm soooo sorrrrry!'"

Survival became Kryszak's focus, and that meant taking care of the gear she needed to pull her through bad situations. Her truck was in good shape, and it meant safety. When someone else used it, she felt increasingly in danger and increasingly angry.

That was the case one morning when she was ordered to go to a nearby hill with two antennas to serve as a relay point for messages from forward observation base Scania to their base camp, FOB Kalsu. Her truck had been taken by an earlier relay team, leaving her with a truck with a weak battery; she had a bad feeling about it. "I was angry because I really didn't want to be there," she said. "I threw my Kevlar [helmet] on the ground, walked away, and sat down by one of the Humvees."

For about a quarter of an hour, it was quiet. Then there was a tremendous explosion. "We all ran for a little makeshift bunker. You could hear the mortars being launched, so you knew they were close. We were getting mortar fire from two sides and some small arms fire. I looked at my friend and said, 'Dude, I don't want to die here.' He said, 'We're not going to die here,' and then he hugged me for about 30 seconds. Then all the adrenaline kicked in, and we jumped up and saw all the incoming fire. I realized there was no one on the radio calling for help, so I got on the radio and called for reinforcements. By the time they got there, we were still taking a lot of incoming fire. We realized we had to get out of there, so I got into the truck with the bad battery, and it started. It started! But then the other truck wouldn't start, so in the middle of that firefight, I'm standing out in front of the two Humvees holding battery cables and trying to jumpstart that truck."

When it finally started, they jumped on board and flew down the hill between the mortar positions. "Once we got out of there, I said, 'I'm never going back there! I can't go back there! You can't make me go back there!'" When the trucks got back to the base camp, Kryszak was ordered to brief the commanding officers on what had happened on the relay hill. "And when I got back from that, all I could do was sit on the floor and cry and cry and cry," she said. "Because it was at that moment that I knew I could have died, that I'd never go home."

Being home wasn't enough

But Kryszak did come home. She was elated to begin with, then discovered that things weren't right with her. Depression began to keep her in her room. "And I began to notice that my temper was really short. I couldn't wait in the checkout line in the grocery store. Little things that shouldn't bother me — my college roommate not putting the dishes away — really, really bothered me. Once my boyfriend went to visit a friend, said he'd call and didn't. He was just having too much fun and forgot. But I got really upset, threw my cell phone, and punched a hole in the wall. At that point, I realized something was wrong with me."

Kryszak thought she'd shake the depression when she graduated from the State University of New York in Buffalo, got a new job, and moved to Chicago. But the relief was brief, far too brief. She found, for instance, that she couldn't handle taking a train to work. "If the trains were too crowded, I couldn't get on. I'd start to hyperventilate, and I couldn't make myself get on. I'd wait for four or five trains before I found one I could board. Then I had to be in a position where my back was in a corner and I could see everyone. Even now, I don't like things behind my back that I can't see. When the train went underground, I began counting down the seconds before it would blow up. Every day that happened. I was so used to IEDs that I couldn't stop myself from counting down until the explosion. Then when I got off the train, I'd walk the rest of the way to work using a different route every day because I was worried that people would pick up on a routine."

Kryszak was working with a children's multimedia entertainment company based in Chicago, and she tried to talk about her problems. To her relief, her co-workers were supportive, helpful, and understanding. When someone noticed she was stressing out, they'd suggest a walk or another diversion to break the mood.

But some things are huge triggers. The smell of diesel fuel takes her back to Iraq immediately and makes her nauseated. And she completely lost it on her first Fourth of July back in the states. "We were coming back from a party because I wanted to get home before the first fireworks started. We were walking down the street, and everyone had these mortar fireworks. They were going up and going off, and I dropped to the ground immediately and started crying. The worst sound they make is when they launch. As many times as I've been mortared in Iraq, it's enough to cause instant panic attacks. I was running to our house, crying. I've heard that *whump* when infantry guys in our base camp set off their flares. I've never experienced such instant panic, where my insides were knotting up and balling up. You tighten up and crouch like you're in pain, and it doesn't go away until the fireworks stop," she said.

Kryszak's flashbacks are relatively minor — she can usually shake them off in a second or two — but the nightmares are ugly. "The nightmares are usually about getting hit by IEDs in our vehicles or when I was up on the relay hill getting mortared," she said. "At that time, no one was injured badly, but in my dreams, the people I really care about keep getting hurt. It gets progressively worse, and I have no control, no way of stopping it. When I wake up, I'm sweating and my heart is pounding."

Kryszak used to get those dreams two or three times a week. Now they're just as intense, but two or three times a month. "I don't know whether it's the medications I'm on or the therapy or just the passage of time," she said. "And I really don't care. I just want to get through this. If it's working, I don't want to change it."

Rooting out bad memories

Practitioners of Eye-Movement Desensitization and Reprocessing believe that most psychopathologies are rooted in early life experiences and that they must be transformed into positive things by incorporating positive insights and affects and removing self-denigrating memories.

Francine Shapiro, the founder of EMDR, said she discovered the new methodology in 1987 as she was dealing with some unsettling thoughts of her own. As she gauged her own reactions to them, she realized that her eyes began to move very rapidly back and forth in an upward diagonal as the memories afflicted her. Later when the thoughts returned, the emotional charge that they brought with them was much less, so she began to focus on eye movement as a way of removing the emotional charge from her memories. As she began to move her hands in front of patients' faces and ask them to focus on her fingers, she said she found she could replicate her own success in others. Over the next six months, she worked with about 70 patients and essentially developed a standard procedure that consistently reduced their complaints.

Her procedure assumes that pathological memories contain dysfunctional information that is physiologically stored and can be accessed without the use of medication. Rather than going after the reaction to the memory, EMDR goes after the memory itself, which usually has emotional components — picture, cognition, affect, and physical sensations. A successful treatment can bring out those memories, strip them of their emotional content, and store them away again in a less threatening form. Shapiro's belief is that the normal information processing system has been blocked part way through, but that reprocessing the memory completes the process. Along the way, the patient's sense of self-worth and self-efficacy are restored. And it can happen fairly quickly. Shapiro said controlled studies have shown that

77-90 percent of civilian PTSD cases can be resolved with three 90-minute sessions.

Shapiro said one of her early patients was a Vietnam vet who had served as an infantryman during his tour of duty in the 1960s. One of his duties was unloading dead bodies from a rescue helicopter. Shapiro said she asked him to hold that memory in his mind while he followed her hand with his eyes. As he did, she said, portions of the image began losing their power until his memory looked like "a paint chip under water." He felt calm enough to go home and help other vets, said Shapiro, and he has remained that way.

Since then, controlled studies have shown EMDR brought a marked decrease in flashbacks, nightmares, and other PTSD symptoms to soldiers serving in Desert Storm, the Vietnam War, the Korean War, and World War II. One EMDR study with combat vets who received a full 12 sessions showed 78 percent no longer suffered PTSD symptoms after treatment or after nine months.

Shapiro stresses two basic themes in dealing with vets. The first is that no one is as bad as they really think they are; if they were, they wouldn't be suffering. And the second is that agonizing over past events doesn't help those who suffered in the past, but it does block a vet from doing anything worthwhile in the present.

One major fear is a loss of self-control. Combat is something that no one can control, and vets fear being back in that chaos. Consequently, they have a strong need to control their own destinies. That's even more true after years in which they are victims of their own disorder. So it's important that they realize that they must be strong enough to accept that there are things outside all of our control.

Vets are also unsettled when they go into treatment to cure combat-related problems and discover that issues of childhood trauma begin to surface. Remember our previous discussion about the poverty draft? Many soldiers joined the military because they hoped it would take them away from the civilian traumas they had been facing. If they were neglected as children, traumatized by alcoholic parents, or abused sexually, war experiences may well bring out these previous traumas. And even though they appear to be secondary to the combat trauma, these underlying issues can't be ignored.

Another peril is that a known demon may be less threatening than an unknown one. Veterans may fear that they'll lose some important things during treatment. They may fear losing: 1) their identification as warriors; 2) their reliance on wartime trauma as a justification for years of post-service failure; or 3) the constant vigilance that saved their lives on the battlefield (who knows if they'll need that skill again?). Finally, recovery can be a threat if it threatens a VA disability check and the vet has no other marketable skill.

Fear of forgetting is particularly unsettling. A vet needs to understand that losing his pain does not mean he'll never remember his combat experience or the people who went through it with him. And he needs to understand that living a healthier and happier life will give him or her more opportunities to help others. Sometimes, post-treatment service to other veterans or to the widows and children of fallen comrades will offer vets a renewed sense of self-worth. Since that combat bonding is a part of all vets, it's important to hold a group together when some begin to feel alienated from the rest because some are forging ahead while others are falling behind.

Emotional Freedom Techniques

Gary Craig, a Stanford engineer who is neither a psychologist nor a trained therapist, has developed a treatment called Emotional Freedom Techniques (EFT) that's similar in some ways to EMDR. It's based on the theory that imbalances in the body's energy system have profound effects on a person's physical and mental health, and that tapping on certain points on the body can quickly correct those imbalances.

According to Craig, EFT removes some of the unnecessary complications of an earlier set of techniques called Thought Field Therapy (TFT) developed by Roger Callahan. There have been a few controlled studies reported in scientific journals including one in the *Journal of Clinical Psychology* by Wells and others that demonstrated EFT's success in reducing phobias. However, EFT is new enough that most of the evidence comes from therapists' observations or reports by people who have experienced EFT.

The best major study is an audit and preliminary trial of TFT and EFT techniques on 29,000 patients, including 5,000 with anxiety disorders, in Uruguay. According to the *South American Studies: Summary and Discussion of Clinical Data*, "No reasonable clinician, regardless of school of practice, can disregard the clinical responses that tapping elicits in anxiety disorders (over 70 percent improvement in a large sample in 11 centers involving 36 therapists over 14 years)."

Closer to home, Dawson Church, director of research for the Association for Comprehensive Energy Psychology, reported in an unpublished manuscript about a study of 11 veterans and their families to treat PTSD and other conditions. Church concluded: "Therapists reported that while they were able to facilitate resolution of most of the combat-related traumas during the course of five days, they were not able to address all the other issues in the participants' lives."

There are a lot of theories about why therapies like EFT work. Michael Lamport Commons of the Department of Psychiatry at the Harvard Medical School suggests that these therapies are "working at the subcortical level of brain activity to interrupt the negative emotional responses elicited by the trauma stimuli." He goes on to suggest that PTSD reactions overwhelm any other kind of mental or emotional processing in the brain. Some aspects of EFT, and he is not certain exactly which they are, break the strength of the PTSD reaction and allow healing to take place.

Phil Mollon, a British psychiatrist, also concludes that the various activities disrupt the intensity of the traumatic memory. In another unpublished paper, he wrote, "At certain points, the tapping is accompanied by eye movements, humming and counting — a constellation of multisensory activities that appears to increase the disruption of the cognitive-emotional response." Others have suggested that the tapping, eye movements, humming, and counting provoke release of serotonin in the prefrontal cortex and amygdala which mitigates the imaginal activation of the fear response.

Craig, himself, points to the 5,000-year-old Chinese insights into the human energy system including those used in acupuncture. The Chinese used acupuncture to correct energy imbalances by sticking a very small needle into energy circuit centers and twirling the needle. Many modern acupuncturists no longer actually puncture, but use a small tingle of electricity to remove blockages. There is also a school of acupressure that treats pain by applying pressure to a convergence of nerves. For example, a headache can be relieved by pressing on a spot in the forehead right above the bridge of the nose. Craig believes you can do the same thing by tapping those points. "By simply tapping near the end points of your energy meridians, you can experience some profound changes in your emotional and physical health," he wrote in his *EFT Manual*. Although the memory of a trauma remains, the emotional charge and the fear disappear.

Linda Geronilla, a West Virginia counselor whom I've known and trusted for a quarter century, is running a national pilot study on EFT on veterans at Marshall University in Huntington. "Most of the trauma resides in the amygdala," she told me. "Energy therapies use the meridian lines honored in China. We tap on the line at its end point. It's like tapping a violin string — when you touch it, the whole thing vibrates. When you touch the end points of this meridian line, particularly the points on the face, it directly affects the amygdala."

Perturbed by the high cost and low effectiveness of American medicine, Geronilla began looking to other cultures and was attracted to the Chinese model. She was particularly pleased that it didn't involve medications. "This relaxes a part of the brain that has been traumatized," she explained. "Then the parasympathetic nervous system can relax, and the heart rate and blood pressure both go back to normal."

She has just finished a study involving nine vets on campus, of whom five received EFT treatment. While the study size was small, she said all showed improvement that appears to be long-term.

One of those participating in the study was Cory Payne, faculty advisor to the student vets association at Marshall University. A medical discharge in 2004 ended his 18-year career in the Army, and later the National Guard. Iraq was his eighth and final deployment. "Bosnia was the toughest," he told me. "It was an ethnically divided region, and our interpreters were all people who had fought against each other. It was horrible. Our interpreters told us about and showed us mass graves. We had explosions in our compounds. The amount of atrocities that went on in that region were enough to rattle you. I stopped at an orphanage and saw all the kids with missing limbs whose families were dead or couldn't take care of them. Then there was the Persian Gulf, the burned bodies and all that devastation. It all took its toll on me. It turned me into an alcoholic for quite a while."

Common cooking smells — and particularly barbequing — made him gag, choke, and vomit three and four times a day. But the EFT therapy has provided him with relief, Payne said. "EFT focuses on certain parts of the body that you're stimulating, and you're training your mind to think of one item each session. I would think about vomiting, for example. We would introduce that smell, and all I could think was that I wanted to go outside and have a cigarette. So Linda would say to me, 'Concentrate on the smell of the cigarette.' Eventually the smell of my Marlboro took away the smell of burning flesh, and now it has replaced the trigger of my vomiting. I just wish I could do something about my smoking."

Since 1997, Payne said he has slept only two or three hours a night because nightmares would wake him up in a panic and send him running for the commode. "But I'm sleeping five hours a night now, something I haven't done in 10 years," he said. "Last night, I had a nightmare and woke up with the night sweats, but no vomiting.

"I think it's awesome," Payne told me. "I just wish the Army and the VA would use it. The VA is the biggest pharmaceutical company going, and that's wrong. We have a lot of vets at Marshall going through the day so doped up they can hardly think. I've seen a number of news stories about vets in trouble, vets taking the drugs that no longer work and getting depressed and doing something stupid. That's why I don't like taking the meds. And that's why I am forever in Linda's debt for helping me with EFT."

Geronilla is now gearing up to run a bigger national pilot program, one that will involve about 10 clinicians and 100 patients in Huntington.

For veterans who have PTSD it really doesn't matter why it works. The real advantages to EFT are that it seems to work on PTSD for some people and that the veteran can try the technique for himself without waiting for an appointment with a practitioner. For difficult problems such as PTSD it is often easier to get successful results with the help of an EFT practitioner, but many people have reported good effects doing EFT on their own.

Another advantage is that it does not require dwelling on the devastating memories. "There is relatively little emotional suffering involved with EFT," says Craig. "It is relatively painless. You will be asked to briefly recall your problem — there may be some discomfort in that — but that is all. There is no need to relive the pain. In fact, with EFT, generating prolonged emotional discomfort is frowned on."

Although it may be possible to isolate a complaint and specify which points need to be tapped, Craig believes it's often easier just to go for a 100 percent overhaul. He said tapping points that are operating normally does no harm.

For Payne, tapping is quickly soothing. "I can feel my heart rate lowering," he said. "I feel like a kid lying in bed, and I can fall asleep immediately. I can do a set of four tappings and then, no matter what time of the day it is, I can lie down and sleep like a baby."

In the summer of 2008, Gary Craig announced that he and five EFT experts did an intensive therapy with 11 veterans and their family members. They gathered data on their levels of PTSD before and after the event and found that those levels dropped by an average of 63 percent. "We've followed their progress for the last three months, and they've maintained most of the ground they gained," Craig said.

Now, the Iraq Vets Stress Project, which offers EFT to all veterans free of charge, is launching a nationwide study of vets with PTSD (whether or not they served in Iraq). There is more information at http://www.StressProject.org for anyone who is interested in participating.

EFT Techniques

The full description of how to do EFT is available at no cost on Craig's website, www.emofree.com. This summary shows some of the basic ideas. Before you start, rate your level of discomfort on a scale of zero to ten, where zero is no discomfort and ten is as much as you can stand. No one who does EFT will be surprised if you rate yourself well over ten on this scale.

The first thing is to make sure you have no "polarity reversal," a situation that Craig said is akin to putting batteries backward into an appliance. It's caused by self-defeating, negative thinking that must be reversed before any improvement can occur. You can do this by mentioning your problem as specifically as you can, then saying something positive about yourself three times.

For Kryszak, that might be, "Although I have terrible nightmares about not being able to start our trucks during the mortar attack, I deeply and completely love and accept myself." This affirmation is said while the patient: 1) vigorously rubs one of two spots on their upper chest a couple of inches above the nipples (called the sore spots because that's where lymphatic congestion occurs); or 2) vigorously taps what's called the karate chop point, the fleshy part of the outside of your hand between the wrist and the baby finger. Either of these procedures may take ten seconds or less.

Then Craig would have you begin the tapping sequence. There are two ways to go through the sequence: a short form and a long form.

The short form is usually enough and is much less complicated. You say a reminder phrase about the problem ("terrible nightmares") and tap about seven times on each pressure point. Five of them are on your face: the base of your eyebrow, the bone bordering the outside corner of the eye, the bone about an inch below your pupil, the area between your nose and your upper lip, and midway between your lower lip and your chin. Three are on your torso: one where your breastbone, collarbone, and first rib meet (about an inch down from the knot of a man's tie and another inch left or right); the second on the side of the body parallel with a man's nipple or in the center of a woman's bra strap; the third about an inch below a man's nipple or at the point where the lower part of a woman's breast meets her chest wall. Then go through the points again.

In the long form you add the following points. Tap on five points on your hand: the outside edge of your thumb even with the base of your thumbnail; the outside edge of your index finger, again even with the base of the nail; the same place on your middle finger; the inside of your baby finger, again at the base of the nail; and the karate chop point mentioned above.

Note that each of these points is mentioned in descending order to make it easier to remember.

Here's where the long form begins to resemble EMDR, but also where it becomes even trickier. Craig has isolated what he calls the Gamut point, which is on either hand half an inch behind the midpoint between the knuckles of the ring finger and the little finger. Between the two sets of tapping on points on the body, tap the Gamut point continuously and perform these nine actions in sequence: 1) close your eyes, 2) open your eyes, 3) look hard down to the right while holding your head steady, 4) look hard down to the left while holding your head steady, 5) roll your eyes in a circle around the perimeter of your vision, 6) do the same thing in reverse, 7) hum two seconds of a happy song like "Happy Birthday," 8) count rapidly from one to five, and 9) hum two seconds of the happy song again.

As with the short form, run through the 13 tapping points one more time, including the reminder phrase ("terrible nightmares") with each point. That tells your system which problem needs to be corrected, according to Craig.

When you are through, check your level on the zero to ten scale again. If it's down, but not to zero yet, go through the tapping sequence until you get it to zero (or as low as you can). Be aware that you can shift from one aspect of the problem to another — this is normal — and try to rate the specific incident you started with rather than the new aspect (usually a new memory) that has emerged. It will give you a better feel for your progress.

If that all sounds too confusing, check out the EFT website (www.emofree.com). Craig will let you download a manual with diagrams of the tapping points or ask for a physical copy. He also has videos available that demonstrate the proper actions in the proper sequence that you can follow. Practitioners have also provided descriptions of how they use EFT for PTSD.

Craig described EFT in a nutshell: "Memorize the basic recipe listed above. Aim it at any emotional or physical problem by customizing it with the appropriate setup affirmation and reminder phrase. Be specific where possible and aim EFT at the specific emotional events in one's life that may underlie the problem. Where necessary, be persistent until all aspects of the problem have disappeared. Try it on everything!!"

And he said there's a generalization principle. If you have a number of specific problems and begin treating them one by one, fairly soon they all disappear. "Some people (like war veterans) have hundreds of traumatic memories," Craig wrote in his *EFT Manual*. "If you are among them, you can expect the generalization effect to work for you. For example, if you have 100 traumatic memories, you probably need to address only about 10 or 15 of them. After that, you are likely to have difficulty getting any emotional intensity over the remaining ones. The generalization effect will have neutralized them."

Church, who is also executive director of the Soul Medicine Institute in Fulton, California, can't explain the phenomenon, but has seen it work. "I certainly do believe in the power of the human electromagnetic field to shift cellular function," he wrote me. "But it's not a mystical effect; it's simply an under-researched aspect of biology. One of the reasons that the energy explanations have been favored is that traumatic memories lose their emotional charge in compressed time frames, frames so brief that they seem like miracles and boggle the mind. But since these traumas were laid down in seconds, why not posit a healing mechanism that extinguishes them in seconds?"

- 21 -
Conclusions

We need to reduce the pain, anxiety, and anger from our Faces of Combat, but, as a nation, we haven't done a very good job treating PTSD and TBI. Here are some of my thoughts about how we should improve.

War should not be entered into lightly because the costs of war are enormous. But America has been in a series of almost unbroken conflicts for the past two generations, virtually since we got sucked into Vietnam 40 years ago. By 2008, America had deployed 1.6 million men and women to Iraq and Afghanistan, including 1.1 million in the Army Reserves and the National Guard, often on two and three deployments. The price of our current war will be huge in shattered men (and now women) and in their medical bills.

The aftermath of war is not something one thinks of when battle plans are bring drawn, but we must think of it because we owe ongoing care to the soldiers injured in service to their country.

For all our recent wars — from World War II to Korea to Vietnam to the dozens of "peace-keeping missions" to Iraq — that cost is beyond calculation. But Linda Bilmes, a professor of public finance at the John F. Kennedy School of Government at Harvard University, and Joseph Stiglitz, a Columbia University professor who won the 2001 Nobel Prize for economics, say this war will end up costing America $5 trillion.

What's $1 trillion? In the United States and France, it's considered to be one thousand billion, a one followed by 12 zeroes. It's a little more than the entire U.S. government spends in a single year. And that cost would increase our national debt by about 11 percent, from $9 trillion to $10 trillion.

One major expense is medical care by the Veterans Affairs department for 1.4 million returning veterans at the time of the analysis by Bilmes and Stiglitz. If all troops were withdrawn by 2010 and expenses continued for another 20 years, it would cost us $69 billion. If troops continue to be deployed until 2015 and those costs continue through the 40-year lifetime of the veterans, those costs could be $144 billion.

An additional cost is traumatic brain injuries and post-traumatic stress disorder, the two signature injuries of the current war. The economists estimated that about 20 percent of those injured in Iraq have suffered head/brain injuries that will require a lifetime of care at a cost ranging from $600,000 to $5 million. That will add an additional cost of $14 billion to $35 billion, depending on the length of the conflict and the soldiers' lives.

Soldiers wounded in combat — and National Guard troops automatically became eligible as soon as they were deployed into combat — get disability pay. At current rates, that figures out to an annual payment of $2.3 billion a year. Depending again on the duration of the conflict and the soldiers' longevity, that could range from $53 billion to $87 billion.

When it first was issued, the Bilmes-Stiglitz report pegged the direct costs at $1 trillion, with indirect costs about the same. That $2 trillion estimate drew widespread criticism as being way too exaggerated, but a year later, the nonpartisan Congressional Budget Office said the Bush administration had already spent $600 billion on the War against Terror, 12 times the original $50 billion estimate. It increased projections of the war's probable costs to $2.4 trillion. That's about $8,000 for each American man, woman, and child. The CBO based its estimates on Bush administration projections that the United States could remain mired in the war until 2017 and that it is fighting the war on borrowed money. It projected that interest costs could total more than $700 billion over the course of the war.

By early 2008, Stiglitz and Bilmes had realized their estimates were way too low, particularly since the entire war is being financed with borrowed money and no one thought to include the cost of interest.

"The bottom line is that to the extent the spending is not offset by higher taxes or reduced spending elsewhere in the budget, and therefore simply adds to the deficit, the total budgetary impact of the war, including spending to date, possible future spending, and higher interest costs would amount to between $1.7 trillion and $2.4 trillion through 2017," said Peter Orszag, the head of the CBO.

"To put it all on our credit cards with no accountability, no plan to pay it back, I think is the height of irresponsibility," said Rep. James McGovern, D-Massachusetts, an outspoken war critic who serves on the budget panel. "It will be just one more toxic legacy of this disastrous war we will have to leave our kids to clean up."

After the Persian Gulf War in 1991, half of the soldiers sought VA medical care and 44 percent of them filed for disability benefits. If that continues to hold true in this war, American taxpayers could shell out between $300 billion and $600 billion, depending on how long the war lasts and how long the soldiers live, according to Bilmes and Stiglitz.

So the duo bumped their cost estimate for the war up to $3 trillion to $5 trillion. "America is a rich country," Stiglitz, former World Bank chief economist and a professor at Columbia University, told the congressional Joint Economic Committee. "The question is not whether we can afford to squander $3 trillion or $5 trillion. We can. But our strength will be sapped... There is no such thing as a free war."

By the end of 2007, America's national debt was expanding by about $1.4 billion a day, or nearly $1 million per minute. That left every American man, woman, and child with a debt of about $30,000. And owing a mind-numbing $9.13 trillion, the United States won't be able to make interest payments on that debt, which stood at $5.7 trillion when President Bush took office and is projected to nearly double to $10 trillion by the time he leaves office in January 2009. In 2006, the federal government paid $430 billion in interest on our debt.

"This is the first war ever that's been totally financed by borrowing, by deficits," said Stiglitz. "Because we haven't raised taxes, because we've tried to pretend that this war is for free, we've been skimping on our treatment of veterans."

And things will only get worse. Over the next 25 years, the number of Americans aged 65 and older is expected to double with huge increases in the amount of Social Security and Medicare benefits paid out at the same time that the number of working Americans — workers who pay taxes — will shrink proportionately. There's no money in reserve for that, only debt. That will put huge new demands on an already overloaded system.

"Our estimate is that the national debt will hit 350 percent of the GDP (gross domestic product) by 2050 under unchanged policy," said David Wyss, chief economist at Standard and Poor's, a major credit-rating corporation. "Something has to change because if you look at what's going to happen to expenditures for entitlement programs after us baby boomers start to retire, at the current tax rates, that doesn't work."

The way I figure it, a government with $2 trillion in annual spending and $10 trillion in debt is kind of like a guy who makes $200,000, but who is $1 million in debt. Just for the heck of it, I asked Tom Jacobson, executive director of the Consumer Credit Counseling Service, to run me some figures. He said that if this guy had a $750,000 mortgage at seven percent interest, he'd be paying $4,990 a month over the next 30 years. That's $59,880 a year.

Let's assume he dropped another $250,000 on toys — motor homes and motorboats and the like — and he's taken out a second mortgage to pay that off. If he can even get a second mortgage, it's likely to charge him 12 percent interest. And he needs to pay it off in four years so he can buy new toys. That'll cost him $6,580 a month. That's another $78,960 a year, which brings his annual debt load to $138,840.

That's a deep hole, and it reminds me of the wisdom of the First Law of Holes: "When you're in a hole, quit digging." That interest is the killer. Over 30 years, this guy will pay back the million he owes, plus more than $1.6 million in interest alone. That's not the way I run my household, and it's not the way I would choose to run my government.

While our government is dealing with lower interest rates on its debts, I submit that the principle is the same. We're going to have a very difficult time just paying for Bush's war, not to mention the human aftermath.

In fact, we pay five times more in interest than we spend on the Veterans Administration — five times more than we spend to treat our vets with traumatic brain injuries or post-traumatic stress disorder that they suffered defending our country. President Bush is proposing to spend $84 billion on the VA in 2008, while the government spends $430 billion paying interest on money we've borrowed, nearly half of it on his watch.

And that's truly irresponsible.

What do we need to do?

I promised conclusions in this chapter, and I think there are at least five major lessons we need to learn, five major reforms we need to make.

The first is election reform. Step back for a second and think about it. The current electoral system is funded by rich businessmen who give buckets of money to politicians so they'll get favors after their candidate takes office. The candidates use the money to buy appealing but vague sound snippets on television, then hop into their jets and bounce around the country making canned speeches, smiling to the television cameras, and avoiding questions. It's a system that panders to the greed, stupidity, and laziness of the American public, and as we've found, it's a system that allows the village idiot to be elected to the nation's highest office.

While it's true that democracy is representative and we elect people like us to do our collective will, I believe a better system — one that limits funding and forces candidates to campaign directly to voters instead of to television ad directors — would allow us to elect better candidates. And that is something we clearly need to do. We cannot again make the mistake of electing a president who bankrupts our nation by sending us into a war based on made-up threats to our national security. Along with the increased reliance on democracy, of course, comes the responsibility of an electorate to learn the issues and participate in the process.

Second, we need fiscal responsibility. Where was Congress, the keeper of the nation's checkbook, when America launched a war under false pretences that has cost us tens of thousands of lives and perhaps up to $5 trillion in debt? (See Comment No. 1 about election reform and the village idiots.) We also need a Congress that lives up to its responsibilities to the nation and to its constituents, not to the donors who finance their elections. With a few exceptions, this gutless group of legislators has been a disgrace.

Third is that war should be defensive only. We have no business invading other countries without cause. I think we can defend ourselves if America is under attack and we're forced to go to war. But we should boost our taxes and cut consumer spending to pay for it. We should also impose a new draft instead of hiring mercenaries to do a big chunk of our fighting. If these measures aren't popular, then it means the threat isn't severe enough to go to war. Around the rest of the world, America is perceived as a bully. That's because we've forgotten that other nations have a right to run their own affairs, just as their own citizens have a right to rebel if those affairs are mismanaged. We cannot and should not intervene unless the United States — not Shell Oil, IBM, or Ford Motor Co. — is directly threatened.

Fourth, we must recognize that the costs of war go beyond mere casualty counts. As a number of former soldiers have told me, man was not designed to kill each other. I turn to the Bible, which contains some of the most radical and remarkable insights that I know, and I read of Jesus telling his disciples that two of the Ten Commandments summarize them all: Love the Lord your God with all your heart and soul, and love your neighbor as yourself. The message of the New Testament is love. We should be helping the rest of the world resolve their problems, not invading their countries and killing their residents. Perhaps if we spent half the money currently budgeted for the Department of Defense and used it to provide infrastructure and schools and medical assistance for developing nations, we would find that we didn't need our military forces as often.

And *last*, Montana is beginning to set an example of how to help our returning warriors. It involves recognizing that they're going to come home with injuries, both physical and emotional, and we owe them help with both. It's obvious that we need to build ramps to accommodate vets in wheelchairs, but it's less obvious that we need to provide equal help to vets with invisible injuries: post-traumatic stress disorder and traumatic brain injury. We learned that lesson from Chris Dana's death on March 4, 2007, and the reforms that followed have been remarkable. Assessing our soldiers more closely and for a longer period of time is hugely important. So is helping them readjust to a civilian world and to their families again. So is a system of crisis response teams to be alert for kids who may be falling through the cracks, isolating themselves from their families and buddies because they're too depressed or stressed out to function.

Perhaps the most important part of this reform is its extension to veterans of all eras. As we're beginning to discover, the Vietnam War vets came home to a nation angry at the war and angry at them. Most of them got no help and have been suffering ever since. That was wrong. As the Montana National Guard wisely decided, that must never happen again. All vets injured fighting for their country deserve our compassion and our help.

My fervent hope is that these reforms become the first steps in getting vets across the nation the help they deserve. I hope you will join my protest to improve treatment for our veterans. To get started sign up now on FacesOfCombat.US.

Where to Get Help

For immediate or emergency assistance, please call: The National Veterans Foundation at 1-888-777-4443 or the VA Suicide Prevention Hotline at 1-800-273-8255. Both hotlines are free and confidential.

General

The Department of Veterans Affairs

Find out about health and education benefits, employment assistance, home loans, life insurance, pensions, and memorial services for veterans. Plus special information for minorities and women in the military, and services for homeless and disabled vets.

web: www.va.gov
VA benefits: 1-800-827-1000
Education: 1-888-442-4551
Health Care: 1877-222-8387

The American Legion

The American Legion was chartered by Congress in 1919 as a patriotic, mutual-help, wartime veterans' organization. A community-service organization, The American Legion now numbers nearly 3 million members in nearly 15,000 posts worldwide. Among the resources offered are military family support and service assistance resources.

web: www.legion.org
Veterans Affairs and Rehab: 202-861-2700

National Veterans Foundation
Call their national hotline for veterans seeking resource referral, benefits information, or emotional support.
web: www.nvf.org
phone: 1-888-777-4443

Veterans of Foreign Wars
The Veterans of Foreign Wars has a rich tradition in enhancing the lives of millions through its community service programs and special projects. From providing free phone cards to our nation's active-duty military personnel to raising money for the World War II Memorial, the VFW is there, "Honoring the dead by helping the living."
web: www.vfw.org
phone: 816-756-3390

Iraq and Afghanistan Veterans of America
Founded in June 2004, Iraq and Afghanistan Veterans of America is the nation's first and largest group dedicated to the troops and veterans of the wars in Iraq and Afghanistan, and the civilian supporters of those troops and veterans.
web: www.iava.org/
phone: 212-982-9699 (New York) or 202-544-7692 (Washington, DC)

Vietnam Veterans of America
Founded in 1978, Vietnam Veterans of America, Inc. is the only national Vietnam veteran's organization congressionally chartered and exclusively dedicated to Vietnam-era veterans and their families. VVA is organized as a not-for-profit corporation and is tax-exempt under Section 501(c) (19) of the Internal Revenue Service Code.
web: www.vva.org
phone: 1-800-882-1316

AMVETS
Offers free counseling and claims assistance for honorably discharged veterans and dependants. For almost 60 years, AMVETS has provided service and support to America's veterans and their communities.
web: www.amvets.org
phone: 1-877-726-8387

Blinded Veterans Association
Through service programs, groups, and benefits, BVA promotes the welfare of blinded veterans.
web: www.bva.org
phone: 1-800-669-7079

National Gulf War Resource Center
The National Gulf War Resource Center is an international coalition of advocates and organizations providing a resource for information, support, and referrals for all those concerned with the complexities of Persian Gulf War issues, especially Gulf War illnesses and those held prisoner or missing in action.
web: www.ngwrc.org
phone: 1-866-531-7183

Veterans Service Organization Directory
Check the VA directory for a complete listing of veterans organizations chartered by Congress and/or recognized by the VA for claim representation.
on-line directory: www.va.gov/vso/

Iraq War Veterans Organization
The Iraq War Veterans Organization website has links to information about Veterans Administration health care, readjustment after deployment, education, employment, military discounts, PTSD issues, support-chat forums, family support, and deployment information.
web: www.iraqwarveterans.org

VA Watchdog dot Org
A comprehensive website that provides updated news as well as information about VA benefits, health resources, and political action.
web: www.vawatchdog.org

Stand Up For Veterans
Stand Up For Veterans is a special advocacy campaign of the Disabled American Veterans (DAV). Its purpose is to generate greater public awareness and support for strengthening federal policies that provide assistance to disabled veterans.
web: www.standup4vets.org

Health

National Center for Post-Traumatic Stress Disorder

U.S. Department of Veterans Affairs National Center for PTSD offers a variety of programs as well as resources for education. It publishes numerous journals and answer questions concerning PTSD. The mission of the National Center for PTSD is to provide social services and care to veterans suffering from PTSD and other stress-related disorders.
web: www.ncptsd.va.gov
phone: 802-296-6300

Mental Health Self-Assessment Program

The Mental Health Self-Assessment Program (MHSAP) is a mental health and alcohol screening and referral program provided for military families and service members affected by deployment and mobilization. Anonymous self-assessments are available for depression, bipolar disorder, alcohol use, post-traumatic stress disorder, and generalized anxiety disorder and are offered online, by phone, and at special installations. It is funded by the Department of Defense Office of Health Affairs and coordinated by Screening For Mental Health, Inc.
web: www.mentalhealthscreening.org/military/index.aspx or
www.militarymentalhealth.org
phone: 781-239-0071 or 1-877-877-3647

TRICARE

Find out more about the military managed care system.
web: www.tricare.mil/
phone:　North: 1-877-874-2273
　　　　South: 1-800-444-5445
　　　　West: 1-888-874-9378

NGWRC's Self Help Guide

Great information for those suffering from Gulf War Syndrome, or anyone attempting to file a claim with the VA or Social Security.
web: www.gulfweb.org/bigdoc/selfhelp.cfm
phone: 202-628-2700 ext. 162

Disabled American Veterans

Formed in 1920 and chartered by Congress in 1932, the million-member DAV is the official voice of America's service-connected disabled veterans — a strong, insistent voice that represents all of America's 2.1 million disabled veterans, their families, and survivors. Its nationwide

network of services — free of charge to all veterans and members of their families — is totally supported by membership dues and contributions from the American public. Not a government agency, the DAV's national organization receives no government funds.
web: www.dav.org
phone: 877-I Am A Vet (877-426-2838)

Wounded Warrior Project
The Wounded Warrior Project was founded on the principle that veterans are our nation's greatest citizens. The Project seeks to assist those men and women of our armed forces who have been severely injured during the conflicts in Iraq, Afghanistan, and other hot spots around the world.
web: www.woundedwarriorproject.org
phone: 877-TEAM-WWP

Veterans Eye Care
Launched by the nation's largest group of Eye MDs, VeteransEyeCare.com is a website dedicated to providing quality eye care information and resources for U.S. Veterans.
web: www.veteranseyecare.com

Amputee Coalition of America
This organization, in conjunction with the National Limb Loss Information Center, provides resources for people with limb loss. On its website, you can find parity information for your state, as well as an online support group and a listing for support groups in your area.
web: www.amputee-coalition.org
phone: 1-888-AMP-KNOW (1-888-267-5669)

Blinded Veterans Association
BVA is for those who are a blind or visually impaired veteran, their relatives, or friends. It is an organization specifically established to promote the welfare of blinded veterans.
web: www.bva.org
phone: 202-371-8880

Paralyzed Veterans of America
The PVA Veterans Benefits Department (VBD) provides assistance and representation before the U.S. Department of Veterans Affairs (VA), without charge, to veterans with spinal cord injury and their eligible dependents. They help clients apply for health care, as well as other benefits they are entitled to.

web: www.pva.org
phone: 1-800-555-9140

Lariam Action USA
Lariam Action is an information and support service for people who have questions about the effects of the anti-malaria drug Lariam (mefloquine).
web: www.lariaminfo.org

The Military Vaccine Resource Directory
The Military Vaccine Resource Directory provides an overview of the anthrax vaccine, the latest news, support groups, health care tips, medical, and legal resources for those who are concerned about the military's mandatory bioterrorism vaccines, including the anthrax vaccine. Significant questions have been raised about the effectiveness and necessity of the anthrax vaccine. Reactions to the vaccine include rashes, muscle aches, joint pain, headaches, fever, and nausea. With the vaccine now declared illegal, they work to prevent any further use of investigational new drugs on troops without their informed consent. It also helps the ill and those who have refused the vaccines.
web: www.mvrd.org

Mental Health

Veterans and Families
Veterans and Families is a national non-profit community service and support organization, founded and directed by veterans, parents, grandparents, family members, employers, mental health professionals, academics, and community leaders.
web: www.veteransandfamilies.org
phone: 916-422-5005

National Center for Post-Traumatic Stress Disorder
The National Center for PTSD is a part of the VA that works to advance the clinical care and social welfare of America's veterans through research, education, and training in the science, diagnosis, and treatment of PTSD and other stress-related disorders. Its website is an educational resource concerning PTSD and other enduring consequences of traumatic stress.
web: www.ncptsd.va.gov

Iraq Vets Stress Project

The project offers EFT (Emotional Freedom Techniques) to all veterans free of charge, whether or not they served in Iraq. There are practitioners in many areas of the country and more are joining.
web: www.StressProject.org
phone: 416-922-4325 (project coordinator)

Give an Hour

Give an Hour is a nonprofit organization dedicated to developing a national network of volunteers to respond to acute and chronic needs within our society. It is currently establishing a national network of mental health professionals and reaching out to its first target population, the U.S. troops and families affected by the current military conflicts in Afghanistan and Iraq.
web: www.giveanhour.org

PTSD HelpNet

A practical guide and resource for the troops, vets, and their families who are affected by the pervasive problem of PTSD. The site also offers tips on navigating the VA and seeking professional treatment.
web: www.ptsdhelp.net

Vet Centers

Vet Centers are small community organizations managed by the VA and dedicated to providing counseling *for* combat veterans *from* combat veterans.
web: www.vetcenter.va.gov
phone: 800-905-4675

VVA's PTSD Claims Guide

The purpose of this guide is to assist you, the veteran, or your survivor(s), in presenting your claim for benefits based on exposure to psychologically traumatic events during military service that has resulted in post-traumatic stress disorder (PTSD).
web: www.vva.org/Benefits/ptsd.htm

The Coming Home Project

The Coming Home Project is a non-profit organization devoted to providing compassionate care, support, and stress management tools for Iraq and Afghanistan veterans and their families.
web: www.cominghomeproject.net

Mental Health Self-Assessment Program
MHSAP is a mental health and alcohol screening and referral program provided for military families and service members affected by deployment and mobilization. Anonymous self-assessments are available for depression, bipolar disorder, alcohol use, post-traumatic stress disorder, and generalized anxiety disorder and are offered online, by phone, and at special installations. It is funded by the Department of Defense Office of Health Affairs and coordinated by Screening For Mental Health, Inc.
web: www.mentalhealthscreening.org/military/index.aspx or www.militarymentalhealth.org
phone: 781-239-0071 or 1-877-877-3647

Employment and Job Searches

Hire Heroes USA
Hire Heroes USA is a national non-profit organization, which provides career placement assistance to disabled veterans from Operation Enduring Freedom and Operation Iraqi Freedom. Its mission is to be the bridge to a fulfilling career for our heroes to ensure they have the opportunity to enjoy the freedoms they fought to preserve.
web: www.hireheroesusa.org
phone: 1-866-915-HERO

RecruitMilitary
RecruitMilitary was founded in February 1998 and quickly became a leader in the use of contingency search to place transitioning and veteran personnel in positions in corporate America. RecruitMilitary established its reputation on the basis of unparalleled service, attention to detail in all activities, and great choices for both its job candidates and its employer clients.
web: www.recruitmilitary.com
phone: 513-683-5020

Helmets to Hardhats
Helmets to Hardhats provides the best career opportunities in building and construction trade to those who have earned the nation's support through their years of service and sacrifice, easing the difficult passage into civilian life for military families.

web: helmetstohardhats.org
phone: 866-741-6210

ESGR: Employer Support of the Guard and Reserve
Guardsmen and Reservists have the right to return to their civilian jobs following their service. National Guardsmen and Reservists who think their employers have acted unfairly — for instance, if they believe they were fired because of their military service — should contact the ESGR.
web: www.esgr.org
phone: 800-336-4590

VetBiz
Find out more about starting and running a veteran-owned business.
web: www.vetbiz.gov
phone: 866-584-2344

Veteran Job Search at Military.com
Search over 100,000 job postings online.
web: www.military.com/jobsearch

HireVetsFirst
Veterans seeking employment opportunities can use this free site to search for jobs, get help writing a great résumé, and find out how military skills translate into occupational skills. Employers can also use this site to post job openings.
web: hirevetsfirst.gov
phone: 202-693-4700

REALifelines (Part of HireVetsFirst)
The Recovery and Employment Assistance Lifelines initiative is a joint project of the U.S. Department of Labor, the Bethesda Naval Medical Center, and the Walter Reed Army Medical Center. It will create a seamless, personalized assistance network to ensure that seriously wounded and injured service members who cannot return to active duty are trained for rewarding new careers in the private sector.
web: hirevetsfirst.gov/realifelines
phone: 202-693-4700

Career Command Post
CCP specializes in bringing transitioning active duty military personnel and armed forces veterans together with civilian employers that are

hiring for executive, managerial, professional, technical, skilled, and semi-skilled positions, from the Military Transition Group, Inc.
web: www.careercommandpost.com
phone: 1-800-219-0408

VetJobs.com
A great site for veterans and transitioning military personnel and their family members. Featured are openings for all levels and types of jobs. You can search for jobs (by type, keyword, and location), as well as post your résumé. It is sponsored by Veterans of Foreign Wars of the United States and it's free to job seekers.
web: vetjobs.com
phone: 1-877-VETJOBS

Return to Work
This organization works to provide vocational rehabilitation to veterans returning home from Iraq and Afghanistan. Job seekers and employers can post profiles and connect to help veterans return to work.
web: www.return2work.org
phone: 303-415-9187

Housing

National Coalition for Homeless Veterans
The National Coalition of Homeless Veterans serves to empower homeless veterans so they can support themselves. The NCHV has an excellent page with advice specifically for homeless veterans.
web: www.nchv.org
phone: 800-VET-HELP

U.S. Department of Housing and Urban Development Veteran Resource Center (HUDVET)
HUDVET's goal is to provide veterans and their family members with information on HUD's community-based programs and services. HUDVET is designed especially for homeless veterans to serve as a resource to find housing.
web: www.hud.gov/offices/cpd/about/hudvet
phone: 1-800-998-9999

Department of Veterans Affairs (VA)
The VA has several resources available to homeless veterans. The best way to contact them is by phone. They can provide you with the address and phone number of the VA homeless program coordinator nearest you.
web: www.va.gov
phone: 1-800-827-1000

National Coalition for the Homeless
This organization's mission is to end homelessness. This page points to local organizations for anyone who is homeless or who may become homeless, whether or not they are veterans.
web: www.nationalhomeless.org
phone: 202-462-4822

Education

GI Bill Info from the VA
The official GI Bill Website from the Department of Veterans Affairs.
web: www.gibill.va.gov
phone: 888-442-4551

Federal Student Aid
Federal Student Aid, part of the U.S. Department of Education, ensures that all eligible individuals can benefit from federally funded or federally guaranteed financial assistance for education beyond high school.
web: studentaid.ed.gov
phone: 800-4-FED-AID

The Fund for Veterans Education
The Fund for Veterans' Education was established to provide scholarships to veterans from all branches of the United States Armed Forces who served in Afghanistan or Iraq since September 11, 2001, and who are now enrolled in college or vocational-technical school.
web: www.veteransfund.org
phone: 507-931-1682

Federal Tuition Assistance
The Army Reserve National Guard Federal Tuition Assistance (FTA) Program provides financial assistance to part-time ARNG soldiers in support of their professional and personal self-development goals.
web: minuteman.ngb.army.mil/Benefits/

Legal Assistance

National Veterans Legal Service Program
Provides training and educational publications to help veterans and their dependents obtain all of the benefits that they deserve, and represents veterans and their dependents who are seeking benefits before the U.S. Department of Veterans Affairs and in court.
web: www.nvlsp.org

Military Law Task Force
The National Lawyers Guild Military Task Force assists those working on military law issues as well as military law counselors working directly with GIs.
web: www.nlgmltf.org
phone: 619-463-2369

The Center for Constitutional Rights
The Center for Constitutional Rights (CCR) is a non-profit legal organization dedicated to protecting the rights of those with the fewest protections and least access to legal resources.
web: ccrjustice.org
phone: 212-614-6464.

Board of Veterans Appeals
Find out more about understanding the appeals process.
web: www.va.gov/vbs/bva/

Veterans Consortium Pro Bono Program
The Veterans Consortium Pro Bono Program provides free attorneys to veterans and their qualifying family members who have an appeal pending at the U.S. Court of Appeals for Veterans Claims (Court). If an appellant has filed an appeal with the Court and has been unable to obtain his or her own attorney after 30 days, he or she can request assistance from The Veterans Consortium.
web: www.vetsprobono.org
phone: 1-888-838-7727

ABA Standing Committee on Legal Assistance for Military Personnel
The mission of the ABA Standing Committee on Legal Assistance for Military Personnel is to improve the effectiveness of legal assistance

provided on civil matters to an estimated nine million military personnel and their dependents.
web: www.abanet.org/legalservices/lamp

National Organization of Veterans' Advocates
The National Organization of Veterans' Advocates (NOVA) was incorporated as a non-profit corporation in the District of Columbia in 1993 to serve attorneys and non-attorney practitioners admitted to practice before the U.S. Court of Appeals for Veterans Claims (CAVC). NOVA recognizes the need to share information and analysis in order to provide successful advocacy for veterans. NOVA provides continuing legal education and support to individuals representing veterans.
web: www.navao.org

LawHelp
LawHelp helps low and moderate income people find free legal aid programs in their communities, and answers to questions about their legal rights.
web: www.lawhelp.org

Financial Assistance

Navy-Marine Corps Relief Society
The mission of the Navy-Marine Corps Relief Society is to provide, in partnership with the Navy and Marine Corps, financial, educational, and other assistance to members of the Naval Services of the United States, eligible family members, and survivors when in need. The Society provides interest-free loans and grants, needs-based scholarships, budget counseling, and visiting nurse services, and also operates food lockers and thrift shops.
web: www.nmcrs.org

Army Emergency Relief
AER is a private nonprofit organization incorporated in 1942 by the Secretary of War and the Army Chief of Staff. AER's sole mission is to help soldiers and their dependents.
web: www.aerhq.org
phone: 1-866-878-6378

Air Force Aid Society
The official charity of the U.S. Air Force.

web: www.afas.org
phone: 1-800-769-8951

Coast Guard Mutual Assistance
"We Look after Our Own": Coast Guard Mutual Assistance is a non-profit organization providing financial assistance to the Coast Guard community.
web: www.cgmahq.org
phone: 1-800-881-2462

Military Families

Minstrel Boy
Brian Hart of Bedford, Massachusetts is the blogger of this page. He dedicates it to his late son, PFC John Hart.
web: minstrelboy.blogspot.com

Military Spouse Resource Center
A resource library for military spouse employment, education, and relocation information.
web: www.milspouse.org

National Military Family Association
The NMFA provides timely and useful information to military families.
web: www.nmfa.org
phone: 1-800-260-0218

Sgt. Mom's
Military Life explained by a Military Wife!
web: www.sgtmoms.com

Society of Military Widows
The Society of Military Widows (SMW) was founded in 1968 by Theresa (Tess) Alexander to serve the interests of women whose husbands died: 1) while on active military duty; 2) of a service-connected illness; or 3) during disability or regular retirement from the armed forces. SMW is a nonprofit organization chartered in the State of California under section 501 (c) (4) of the Internal Revenue Service Code.
web: www.militarywidows.org

TAPS (Tragedy Assistance Program for Survivors)
The Tragedy Assistance Program for Survivors, Inc. (TAPS) is a national nonprofit organization made up of, and providing services to, all those who have lost a loved one while serving in any branch of the Armed Forces — Army, Air Force, Navy, Marine Corps, National Guard, Reserves, Service Academies, or the Coast Guard. The heart of TAPS is its national military survivor peer support network. It also offers grief counseling, referral, caseworker assistance, and crisis information, all available to help families and military personnel cope and recover. It provides these services 24 hours a day free of charge.
web: www.taps.org
phone: 800-959-TAPS

VFW National Home for Children
By contacting the VFW National Home for Children, assistance and connection to supportive services nationwide is available to children and families of veterans. In some situations, the children and/or families may be able to become a part of the National Home's campus community where they can live for a time with the opportunity to build a better life. The National Home has four Family Programs to assist families of active duty military members and veterans.
web: www.vfwnationalhome.org
phone: 1-800-424-8360

Women's Issues

Women Veterans Health
The Women Veterans Health Program specifically addresses the health care needs of eligible women veterans, providing appropriate, timely, and compassionate health care at the facility level.
web: www1.va.gov/wvhp

For Women
This website and toll-free call center were created to provide free, reliable health information for women everywhere.
web: www.4woman.gov
phone: 1-800-994-9662

The Miles Foundation
The Miles Foundation has established a toll-free Advocacy Helpline for victims of interpersonal violence associated with the military.

web: hometown.aol.com/milesfdn
phone: 1-877-570-0688

Resources in Your Neighborhood

New Directions
For the past 15 years New Directions has provided comprehensive long-term substance abuse treatment to our nation's veterans. New Directions provides a wide variety of services for homeless veterans, including job training and placement, parenting and money management classes, legal and financial assistance, counseling, remedial education, and resources for alumni.
web: www.newdirectionsbrooklyn.com
phone: 718-398-0800

Swords to Plowshares
This is a non-profit that has been around since 1974, created by Vietnam Veterans to help veterans. It provides housing, legal, employment, and training services, mental health and substance abuse counseling. All their services are free to the veteran and they honor all types of discharges, from honorable to dishonorable. Located in San Francisco, California.
web: swords-to-plowshares.org
phone: 415-252-4788

Veterans Resource Central
Veterans Resource Central (VRC), a Pennsylvania nonprofit organization, provides transition assistance to returning veterans, active duty military and their families through a corps of volunteers and Internet tools. It provides education, information, and guidance to veterans transitioning to civilian life, to military families dealing with life issues at home, and to active duty or recently returned military who are planning their civilian careers.
web: www.veteransresourcecentral.org

Project Healing Waters
Project Healing Waters serves those who have come home wounded. PHW aids in their physical and emotional recovery by introducing or rebuilding the skills of fly-fishing and fly tying.
web: www.projecthealingwaters.org

Medical Glossary

adrenaline — The adrenal glands release adrenaline, also called epinephrine, into the bloodstream under conditions of stress, fear, or excitement. When adrenaline hits the liver, it stimulates the release of glucose for instant energy. Abrupt increases can constrict heart vessels, forcing the heart to pump with higher pressure. It also dilates the pupils of the eyes, constricts arterioles in the skin and the gut, and dilates arterioles in leg muscles to increase human strength, endurance, or agility in an emergency.

amygdala — The brain's flight-or-fight center, the amygdala is an almond-shaped portion in the middle of the brain that is considered part of the limbic system. It's critically important in computing the danger imposed by stimuli, sights, and sounds that it receives through the cortex and smells that it receives directly. It's also involved in computing the emotional significance of events.

cerebrum — The main portion of the brain, about 85 percent of the total, is called the cerebrum and is divided into the left and right hemisphere and subdivided into lobes (frontal, parietal, temporal, and occipital). The top layer of the cerebrum, believed to be the most recent in millennia of evolution, is the cortex.

cortex — Our center of reason, the cortex receives the stimuli from our eyes and ears and passes it along to the amygdala. The frontal lobes of the cortex, located directly behind the forehead, are the center for ethical decision-making, reasoning, planning, reading, and writing. The cortex is what distinguishes us from other animals and makes us human.

cortisol — Manufactured from cholesterol by the adrenal glands, this hormone is produced principally in response to physical or psychological stress. It stimulates the central nervous system, increases water retention and blood sugar for available energy, stimulates the metabolism of proteins to repair injuries, and regulates blood pressure.

dissociation — Trauma can cause the separation of ideas, feelings, information, identity, or memories that would normally go together. It appears to be a normal way of coping with trauma that over time becomes reinforced and develops into maladaptive coping. People say they feel detached from their own feelings, mental processes, or even their own bodies. It can include disassociate amnesia, in which the brain blocks out painful memories.

dopamine — a neurotransmitter, or amino acid, that is normally the body's reward mechanism, rewarding us for doing the things that are good for our body.

fight-or-flight syndrome — One of the oldest human survival tactics, the amygdala weighs the risks and determines whether to confront a danger or run from it. In so doing, it puts the nervous system on high alert, giving it the energy to respond instantaneously.

glucose — A blood sugar, glucose can be added into the bloodstream for instant energy.

hippocampus — This is the memory center of the brain. Its name means "sea horse," based on its shape. The hippocampus is one of the oldest parts of the human brain, another part of the limbic system. It's important in forming and storing associative and episodic memories, including face-name associations, the encoding of traumatic events, and the recall of personal memories in association with smell.

hyperarousal — Caused by hormones triggered by the amygdala, this is the state of imminent fight or flight. It's a white-knuckle, dry-mouth, gut-wrenching, heart-pounding sensation triggered by an immediate threat.

For combat vets with PTSD, it doesn't go away after the threat diminishes or disappears.

hypervigilance — Triggered by memories of past trauma and fears of future threats, PTSD vets go through their days with every sense on high alert. They watch everything, including rooftops, and they mark all the exits and danger zones. Like hyperarousal, it doesn't seem to diminish when the threats subside.

hypothalamus — Located right beside the pituitary gland that produces hormones and working closely with it, the hypothalamus can increase the body's metabolism by releasing a variety of hormones and peptides. The hypothalamus and pituitary gland are part of the autonomic nervous system, which controls such vital body functions as heart and respiratory rate, mental alertness, body temperature, sweating, blood pressure, and pupil dilation.

limbic system — Also known as the mammalian brain, the limbic system governs pain and pleasure, things like fighting, fleeing, eating, and sex. It also appears to play a major role in the storage and retrieval of memories. Damage to two parts of the limbic system, the amygdala or the hippocampus, may cause recurring memories or the loss of the ability to form new memories.

neurotransmitters — Chemicals or amino acids called neurotransmitters pass the electrical currents between cells called neurons in the brain. Dopamine, serotonin, noradrenalin, and the opioids are a few of the most common neurotransmitters that deal with pleasure and pain. All of the brain's normal functions depend on neurotransmitters, and too much or too little of each can lead to serious disorders of thought, mood, and behavior.

serotonin — A neurotransmitter that's been closely related to mood swings and anxiety attacks, as well as regulation of sleep and aggression. Antidepressants like Prozac suppress the absorption of excess serotonin.

Appendix: America's wars

According to Pearson Education, America has had 43.2 million military-era vets, with 1.2 million dying in combat and 1.4 million wounded. We have 18 million living war veterans and 24 million vets total.

Vietnam was America's last major war, but we've had an almost unending series of conflicts recently.

To put it all in perspective, America committed 4.7 million soldiers in World War I, 16.1 million in World War II, and 5.7 million in the Korean War.

In Vietnam, which lasted from 1964 to 1975, America had 8.7 million soldiers, of whom 3.4 million served in-theater. About 90,200 soldiers were killed, 153,300 were wounded, and 7.3 million vets were still living as of 2006, according to the VA.

The Lebanon peacekeeping mission from 1982-84 was much smaller, with 265 American deaths.

In 1983, American forces invaded Grenada in "Operation Urgent Fury" to protect people living there. That resulted in 19 American soldiers killed. The same year, U.S. Marines tried to intervene in a clash between Palestinian refugees and the Lebanese, but 241 Marines were killed when a suicide bomber in a truck carrying six tons of TNT leveled a barracks; seconds later, a second suicide bomber brought down another barracks, killing 58 French troops.

In December of 1989, the United States invaded Panama to oust dictator (and former CIA agent) Manuel Noriega. The death toll for American soldiers was 23.

In 1990-91, America put 2.2 million soldiers into the Gulf War, 665,000 of them in-theater. Nearly 400 died, and another 467 were wounded. There are 1.8 million vets still living.

In 1992, U.S. troops participated in a United Nations peacekeeping mission in Somalia. During a general uprising in Mogadishu, a number of American soldiers were trapped, 19 were killed, and one was filmed being dragged through the streets by an angry mob. Death toll overall: 43.

In the 1990s, American forces were also sent to Macedonia, Haiti, Bosnia for Operation Deliberate Force, the Central African Republic, Albania, the Congo, Sierra Leone, Cambodia, Guinea, Kenya, Tanzania, Afghanistan, Sudan, Liberia, and East Timor.

During the Kosovo War in 1999, America was one of a number of NATO countries that bombed Yugoslavia.

Then in 2001 began the War on Terrorism and Operation Enduring Freedom, the wars that continue to this day with an ever-mounting fatality toll that exceeded 4,000 in the spring of 2008.

Index

More Books from Idyll Arbor and Issues Press

Alcohol: Cradle to Grave

Eric Newhouse

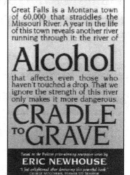

Eric Newhouse, winner of the 2000 Pulitzer Prize for the newspaper columns reprinted in this book, is a veteran newspaper reporter. As such, he's seen the flotsam and jetsam of human life: the divorces, lost jobs, battered wives, abused children, crime, drunken drivers, car wrecks, and medical bills. And, he's come to the conclusion that alcohol is behind much of it. Take away the alcohol and much of the human tragedy goes away.

This book, *Alcohol: Cradle to Grave*, offers a compelling, day-in-the-life look at how the disease of alcoholism affects the state of Montana, as a microcosm of the national problem. Newhouse offers us a compelling and comprehensive understanding of the complexity, magnitude, and cost of alcohol abuse. It's an unflinching look at the largely unnoticed river of booze that is flooding our towns, our communities, and our daily lives — with suggestions on how to channel the flow.

$18.00   Trade paper, 274 pages   ISBN 1-930461-04-6

Outwitting your Alcoholic: Keep the Loving and Stop the Drinking

Kenneth A. Lucas

Foreword by Eric Newhouse

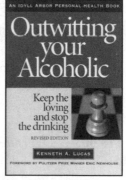

Some people still love their alcoholic partner. They don't want to hear, "Just leave!" They want to find a way to get themselves *and* their loved one out of the trap of alcohol. This book will help readers do that: outwit the alcohol that is ruining their lives.

The world of alcoholism is strange, filled with half truths and whole lies. The journey out of that world can be confusing and difficult, but people have made it. In this book, Ken Lucas provides a map of the alcoholic's world. (He lived there once.) He talks about how to get out, and bring the alcoholic out, too.

$18.00   Trade paper, 208 pages   ISBN 1-882883-60-8

Idyll Arbor Recovery Books

Things That Work: A No-Nonsense Guide to Recovery by One Who Knows
Barry Bocchieri

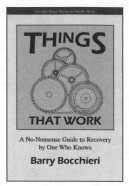

This book is for readers who are beginning to come to terms with their problem. It contains no generalities behind which they can hide, no Pollyanna solutions that will let them believe that they can sidestep the tough times ahead. Instead, they will find the principles that worked for the author in spite of his predisposition for, inclination toward, and background of alcoholism.

$16.00   Trade paper, 140 pages   ISBN 1-882883-61-6

Reflections along the Way: Stories of Recovery and Life from One Who Has Been There
Barry Bocchieri

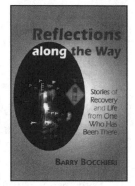

Bocchieri is an expert in the field of substance abuse and addiction. In this book he uses his unique ability of explaining complex psychological, philosophical, and spiritual concepts in clear, concise, and easy-to-understand language to describe how a person can succeed in his or her recovery. This is a more personal follow-up to his first book, *Things That Work: A No-Nonsense Guide to Recovery from One Who Knows*.

$16.00   Trade paper, 142 pages   ISBN 1-882883-66-7